Mosby's

Q&A Review

for the

Occupational Therapy
Board Examination

WITHDRAWN

Mosby's

Q&A
Review

for the

Occupational
Therapy
Board Examination

Edited by

Patricia Bowyer, EdD, OTR/L, BCN

University of Illinois at Chicago
Post Doctoral Research Associate
College of Applied Health Sciences
Chicago, Illinois

Dorothy P. Bethea, EdD, MPA, OTR-L

Chair and Associate Professor
Winston-Salem State University
The School of Health Sciences
Occupational Therapy Department
Winston-Salem, North Carolina

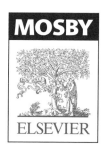

MOSBY

ELSEVIER

11830 Westline Industrial Drive
St. Louis, Missouri 63146

MOSBY'S Q & A REVIEW FOR THE OCCUPATIONAL THERAPY
BOARD EXAMINATION

ISBN-13: 978-0-323-04459-2
ISBN-10:   0-323-04459-X

Notice

Neither the Publisher nor the Authors assume any responsibility for any loss or injury and/or damage to persons or property arising out of or related to any use of the material contained in this book. It is the responsibility of the treating practitioner, relying on independent expertise and knowledge of the patient, to determine the best treatment and method of application for the patient.

The Publisher

ISBN-13: 978-0-323-04459-2
ISBN-10: 0-323-04459-X

Publishing Director: Linda Duncan
Senior Editor: Kathy Falk
Senior Developmental Editor: Christie M. Hart
Publication Services Manager: Melissa Lastarria
Senior Project Manager: Kelly E.M. Steinmann
Designer: Maggie Reid

Working together to grow
libraries in developing countries

www.elsevier.com | www.bookaid.org | www.sabre.org

ELSEVIER   BOOK AID International   Sabre Foundation

Printed in the United States of America.

Last digit is the print number: 9 8 7 6 5 4 3 2 1

Contributors

PATRICIA BOWYER, EdD, OTR/L, BCN
University of Illinois at Chicago
Post Doctoral Research Associate
College of Applied Health Sciences
Chicago, Illinois

DOROTHY P. BETHEA, EdD, MPA, OTR-L
Chair and Associate Professor
Winston-Salem State University
The School of Health Sciences
Occupational Therapy Department
Winston-Salem, North Carolina

SUSAN M. CAHILL, MAEA, OTR/L
Clinical Instructor
Department of Occupational Therapy
University of Illinois at Chicago
Chicago, Illinois

LISA CASTLE, MBA, OTR/L
Director of Occupational Therapy
University of Illinois Medical Center at Chicago
Chicago, Illinois

JENNIFER SUSONG CROWDER, MS, OTR
Occupational Therapist
Sullivan County Department of Education
Blountville, Tennessee

PETER GIROUX, MHS, OTR/L
Associate Professor of Occupational Therapy
University of Mississippi Medical Center
Jackson, Mississippi

CINDY HAHN, MOT, OTR/L, FAOTA
Associate Professor and AMOT Program Director
A. T. Still University
Mesa, Arizona

ANNE E. JENKINS, MA, OTR/L, Ed M
Assistant Professor
Occupational Therapy
Winston-Salem State University
Winston-Salem, North Carolina

BRENDA KORNBLIT KENNELL, BS, MA, OTR/L
Adjunct Professor
Winston-Salem State University
Winston-Salem, NC
Director of Rehabilitation Services
Carolinas Medical Center-Lincoln
Lincolnton, North Carolina

KELLY MILLER LAMBETH, MPH, OTR/L
Senior Occupational Therapist
Wake Forest University Baptist Medical Center
Neurorehabilitation Center
Winston-Salem, North Carolina

JEFF SNODGRASS, PhD, MPH, OTR/L
Program Director and Associate Professor
Occupational Therapy Program
Milligan College
Milligan College, Tennessee

IMOGENE TILSON, MA, OTR/L
Occupational Therapist
Behavioral Health Services
Huntsville Hospital
Huntsville, Alabama

Preface

The intent of this examination guide is to provide a means for strategically preparing for the certification examination. It is important for students to not only understand how the certification examination works, but to implement a plan of action that encompasses review of materials and organization of information into coherent themes or categories, and also to become familiar with test-taking strategies to optimize their performance and test scores. This text is organized to reflect questions in four categories: (1) evaluation, (2) intervention planning, (3) intervention, and (4) administration and service management. This format was selected because these categories are among the major areas that are addressed on the national certification examination for occupational therapy. These areas also are major constructs in comprehending the progression and application of the occupational therapy process. Although each chapter has a central focus, there is a mixture of questions that spans a wide array of diagnoses, populations, and practice settings. While some basic knowledge may be tested, the main idea is for the student to apply knowledge in making rational and good decisions that guide practice.

This text serves as a resource for study purposes only. It is not intended to be the sole source of information or to substitute for other necessary resources, such as course lectures, course textbooks, skilled competencies, and theoretical foundational knowledge, which are all essential to prepare for the certification examination. It may help to identify strengths and areas of need so that the student can focus on a viable plan to prepare for the examination. References used in this text were selected primarily from sources or textbooks that have been identified as being frequently used in occupational therapy educational settings. However, a few references may differ because they provided the best support and rationale to the question. A bibliography is located at the end of the textbook and can provide additional resources from which to study.

Table of Contents

CHAPTER 1

Examination Preparation

When preparing for a board examination, the most effective approach is to closely simulate the behavior you will eventually be required to perform. Advance preparation for the examination is essential and requires both physical and mental stamina and practice. One should practice taking tests in a couple of ways: without accessing your notes to test your knowledge and retention and answering new questions about the same or similar information.

MULTIPLE CHOICE EXAMINATIONS

The national certification examination for occupational therapy is made up of multiple choice questions. Multiple-choice questions generally consist of three parts: (1) a stem, which asks a question, poses a problem, or presents an incomplete sentence; (2) normally one correct answer; and (3) a number of "distracters" or alternatives among which the correct answer is listed. The national certification exam will have four distracters including the correct answer and three likely, but incorrect alternatives. When taking the examination, one should read the question carefully, and then read all the choices before selecting the answer. In some instances, people find it helpful to read the question along with each distracter.

BLOOM'S TAXONOMY

Think of which level in ***Bloom's Taxonomy*** the test is addressing. Most questions on the national certification examination are written at the ***application level,*** meaning that the test taker will need to have basic knowledge and comprehension of the concepts that are being tested and be able to generalize to new situations. The taxonomy is categorized into six levels: knowledge, comprehension, application, analysis, synthesis, and evaluation (see Table).

Level	Explanation	Question Cues
Knowledge	Observation and recall of information, under-standing major ideas and topics	List, define, tell, describe, identify, show, label, collect, examine, tabulate, quote, name, who, when, where, etc.
Comprehension	Understand, interpret information, translate into new context, infer causes and predict consequences	Summarize, describe, interpret, contrast, predict, associate, distinguish, estimate, differentiate, discuss, extend
Application	How information methods, concepts, and theories used to problem solve are in new situations	Apply, demonstrate, calculate, complete, illustrate, show, solve, examine, modify, relate, change, classify, experiment, discover
Analysis	Recognizing patterns and underlying meanings and identifying components	Analyze, separate, order, explain, connect, classify, arrange, divide, compare, select, explain, infer
Synthesis	Using old ideas to create new ones, generalizing facts,see relationships of knowledge in other arenas, draw conclusions	Combine, integrate, modify, rearrange, substitute, plan, create, design, invent, proposes, compose, formulate, prepare, generalize, rewrite
Evaluation	Compare and discriminate between ideas, assess, make choices based on reasoning, verify evidence	Assess, decide, rank, grade, test, measure, recommend, convince, select, judge, explain, discriminate, support, conclude, compare, summarize

The taxonomy provides a structure in which to categorize exam questions. Determining the level of questions that will appear on the exam will enable the test taker to create more appropriate strategies for study and review.

HELPFUL HINTS: PRIOR TO THE EXAM

Initial Plan: Develop a study plan that is well organized and consider study groups to bounce around ideas and information. Know your areas of weakness and focus your resources on strengthening these areas. If you have the option, review grades from the courses that relate to the examination topics. This strategy will help pinpoint areas that need more attention.

Knowledge of Material: Work at understanding the material, because memorization is not enough. Wording of the questions may be different than the way you learned the material. Basic knowledge is only a beginning. Consider different ways of applying the same information. Think of scenarios and use case study examples to demonstrate critical thinking and fully grasp the materials and topics. If you have access to them, study old exams and notes to clear up misconceptions and clarify information.

Predict Questions: Try to predict questions by paying attention to major concepts, theories, study guides, techniques, and review questions at the end of textbook chapters. When you are studying, ask yourself why answers to questions in the text are correct or incorrect.

Time: Set aside time for practice. A good rule of thumb is to try to use the same time and number of questions given during the actual examination. This will increase your comfort level for a similar type of testing process.

The Week Before: The week before the event, get plenty of rest, sleep, and relaxation. Eat well and avoid cramming, because cramming only increases your level of anxiety. Instead, establish a routine and, if you must study, concentrate only on those areas that need clarification. If you established a good plan ahead of time, the likelihood of success is increased.

Testing Center: Identify the nearest testing center where you intend to take your exam. Pay attention to directions and instructions for preparing for the exam, including the location of the site, directions to the facility, arrival time, items required, format of the exam, and instructions that you must adhere to during the actual testing. Bring appropriate documentation and personal identification. Always arrive early at the testing site on the date the examination is scheduled.

Other Options: Examination preparation workshops are sometimes offered and serve as a great review and overview of many subjects. If you have the opportunity, seek out and take advantage of these workshops because they can help students master the materials and concepts needed.

HELPFUL HINTS: DURING THE EXAM

Directions: The occupational therapy certification board examination is computerized. In some instances, a written format of the test can be arranged. Before beginning, you should READ ALL DIRECTIONS CAREFULLY for a clear understanding of the procedures.

Understanding Questions: A good rule of thumb is to try examining each question to determine: (1) the level or type of thinking that is required (e.g., are you required to recognize, analyze, or apply the information presented?) and (2) the degree of difference between the incorrect and correct alternatives.

Ask What, Who, and Why? Consider **what** the question is asking (by paraphrasing), **who** is required to perform (therapist, patient, caregiver), and **why** is one distracter more appropriate to answer the stem (question) than another. Identify key words that could possibly cue you to the best response. For example, is the question asking you to *evaluate, plan, implement,* or *set goals*? Also pay attention to words related to the timing of a particular action, like *initial, first, next*, or *last step*.

Selecting Answers: Do not spend an exorbitant amount of time on questions you truly do not know. Either give your best guess or, if allowed, tag the question and return to it after completion of the exam or of a section of the exam. Use the process of elimination to help you eliminate the obviously incorrect alternatives. Re-read the question for the best fit of the alternative(s) you did not eliminate and then make your selection. Never leave a question unanswered. It is better to guess wrong than to leave an item blank. Check with those giving the examination to find out if there are penalties for marking the wrong answer.

Time: Be cognizant of time, but do not let time be your major focus. Allocate your time according to the relative worth of questions. Try to set a steady but unhurried pace. If possible, save a few minutes at the end for review and revision.

HELPFUL HINTS: AFTER THE EXAM

Relax: People are normally exhausted after taking board exams. Relax for the rest of the day or treat yourself to something special. Talking with fellow students after the examination may help reduce stress. However, do not dwell on the exam or scores.

Results: For the occupational therapy certification exam, test results are sent directly to the candidates within 6 weeks. For a fee, additional requests can be made to send the results to other agencies.

Retesting: Candidates who do not pass the exam on the first attempt can retake it as many time as necessary. There is an application fee each time the exam is repeated, and a 90-day waiting period is required between exams. HOWEVER, WITH DEDICATION AND A THOROUGH PLAN OF ACTION, YOU CAN INCREASE YOUR CHANCES OF SUCCESS!

CHAPTER 2

How to Use this Textbook

Designed as a preparation tool, this textbook can help individuals who are ready to sit for the occupational therapy certification examination, to explore their strengths and weaknesses as they pertain to entry level knowledge about the practice of occupational therapy. Identifying weaknesses may enable individuals to focus their attention and develop strategies that effectively impact the areas of greatest need. The textbook is not designed to replace classroom and field-work education, nor is it meant to be a means for individuals to just memorize or recite answers to questions expecting to pass the certification examination. Instead, this book will allow persons to review general knowledge and target specific areas that they need to focus on while preparing for the certification examination. Furthermore, the CD-ROM offers opportunities to practice com-puterized-based testing, which is the usual format for the certification exam.

University occupational therapy programs provide specific classroom and fieldwork experiences to prepare students to sit for the certification exam, and once the exam is passed, students then have the necessary skills to begin practice as an entry level therapist. In addition, many university programs have found that there is a correlation between students who do well in coursework and those who do well on the certification exam.

Therefore, to best prepare for the certification exam, students should focus on doing well in coursework and then follow that preparation with a specific plan for studying for the certification exam. As part of the preparation, students need to use this text as a guide to help focus study time for the certification exam. Students can use the text to guide them to areas that are weak or in which they have not scored well during their occupational therapy training.

PREPARING FOR THE CERTIFICATION EXAM

1. Determine how and where you will study. Do you study better in a group or alone? If alone, then choose the space you want and need to work in. Set up the area to allow for maximizing your attention. If this requires a quiet, private setting, then find this place in your home environment. If you plan to study with a group, contact those who will participate well in advance of the exam. Organize the location, time,

and subject areas to be reviewed. For some students, a combination of individual study and group study is beneficial. Each person has to determine the best method for developing his or her knowledge in content areas that are weak.

2. Make an honest assessment of knowledge level for any given content area. Through this evaluation process, students are able to acknowledge areas of weakness and in turn focus their study time for the certification exam on strengthening these areas. A way to do this is to review the grades received in courses and review fieldwork evaluations; these are the areas that will require more review in preparation for the certification exam. As part of this review process, use the practice tests in this text to further highlight content areas that require review.

3. Although reviewing materials is vital to gaining content knowledge in areas that are weak, just re-reading course notes may not be enough preparation for the certification exam. Another key aspect to the certification exam is the actual process of taking the exam. The certification exam is computer-based, and because many academic programs do not offer online test taking, this will be the first computer-based exam many students will take. The process for online test taking is different from the process of pencil and paper exams; therefore, students should utilize the CD-ROM provided with this text to practice computer-based testing.

4. When practicing taking the exam, make sure that the environment you practice in will be similar to the environment in which you will take the actual test. In other words, turn off the television, stereo, iPod, or computer and time yourself while taking practice exams. This will help to decrease some of the anxiety that will inevitably occur on the day of the exam. Practicing in an environment similar to that of the actual test will allow you to feel more at ease on the day of the exam because you will have already been through the process.

5. Use the exams in this text as practice exams. Use the same amount of time and number of questions that will be given during the actual exam. This will help prepare you for the amount of pressure in the exam environment.

6. If you can attend a board review session, consider taking it. Sometimes this helps to build confidence about content area that is mastered while helping to further focus areas of need.

CHAPTER 3

Occupational Therapy Practice Framework: Domains and Contents

INTRODUCTION

The Occupational Therapy Practice Framework (AOTA, 2002) is a document that is used to describe the domains of practice for occupational therapy and to outline the process for evaluation and intervention. This document was used to organize this certification review manual. The value of utilizing the Framework as the guide in designing this text is that students are familiar with the Framework from their coursework and the document is designed to provide common terminology to describe the occupational therapy service delivery process.

The practice exams in this text are set up to reflect the Framework language, as are the specific questions included on each exam. The areas that are covered in the practice exams are evaluation, intervention plan, intervention, and service management/administration. These particular process areas were targeted for review within this text because of the results of the National Board Certification for Occupational Therapy (NBCOT) practice analysis. Although students will find each of these broad categories covered in the text, they will also find that populations and practice contexts are covered on each exam.

EVALUATION

The first practice exam covers the area of evaluation. According to the Occupational Therapy Practice Framework (AOTA, 2002), the evaluation process focuses on finding out what a client wants and needs to do. The process involves identifying any factors that are barriers to participation as well as those that support participation. Through this process, the occupational therapist assesses the way in which performance skills impact areas of occupation. The evaluation process determines performance patterns, the context(s) in which they occur, and the demands of an activity, as well as client factors. Once an evaluation has occurred and a determination is made that occupational therapy services are needed, the Framework provides language to discuss the intervention process

INTERVENTION PLAN

The second practice exam covers the area of intervention plan. This area focuses on goal writing, outcomes, and intervention approaches. The intervention plan is the method in which an occupational therapist intends to improve a client's engagement in occupation. The intervention plan is based on the results of the evaluation with input from the client.

INTERVENTION

The third practice exam covers the area of intervention. The area of intervention is the application of techniques to improve engagement in occupation or participation. In this portion of the occupational therapy service delivery process, information from the intervention plan is carried out to improve a client's performance skills as impacted by performance patterns, context, and activity demand and client factors.

ADMINISTRATION AND SERVICE MANAGEMENT

The fourth practice exam covers the area of managing the delivery of occupational therapy services. This portion is not specific to the Occupational Therapy Practice Framework but is included because of the requirements of the certification exam.

Each of the practice exams will include various practice settings and populations with the focus being on the specific domain of evaluation, intervention plan, intervention, and administration/service management. This organization of the practice exams will allow students to focus in on specific content areas that may require in-depth review. The students can use the CD-ROM included with the text to have questions assimilated in a more random manner than is utilized in the layout of the text. It is recommended that a student take advantage of this tool to allow for practice with an exam that will be more in sync with the actual NBCOT exam.

CHAPTER 4

Questions for Evaluation

This practice examination section covers the topic area of evaluation. The questions in this section will relate to the evaluation process, aspects that need to be considered in evaluation, such as diagnoses, client information, and fundamental theories. The primary objective of this practice examination section is to target content knowledge on the overall evaluation process, including screening, the occupational profile, and strategies for selecting, administering assessments, and synthesizing information to guide decision-making. Use this practice examination to determine your knowledge level of the evaluation process.

1. Entry into the early intervention system begins with which of the following?
    a. Screening for developmental delay
    b. Individualized Family Service Plan
    c. Screening for family environmental risk factors
    d. Individualized Education Plan (IEP)

2. In the assessment phase of early intervention, an occupational therapist (OT) assesses the daily living skills of an infant. In the context of early intervention, the areas that are being assessed are:
    a. Feeding and sleeping patterns
    b. Play and leisure patterns
    c. Motor development patterns
    d. Sensory development patterns

3. An assessment team in early intervention has completed an evaluation of a toddler. In compiling the Individualized Family Service Plan, the goals should be determined by the:
    a. Service coordinator for the case
    b. Therapists from each discipline
    c. Reimbursing agency
    d. Parents

4. In early intervention there are different types of risk factors. A child with Down syndrome is an example of:
   a. Biological risk
   b. Environmental risk
   c. Established risk
   d. Recurring risk

5. The parent of a child that is being treated in therapy describes how the child covers their ears when riding in the car with the windows down. The parent does not understand why the child persists in this behavior. The OT explains that this behavior could be the result of:
   a. Sensory defensiveness
   b. Gravitational insecurity
   c. Underresponsiveness
   d. Aversion to movement

6. An OT is using the Peabody Developmental Motor Scales to evaluate a child. The therapist is assessing the child's:
   a. Performance of tasks that support school participation
   b. Visual perception skills in community settings
   c. Gross and fine motor skills
   d. Performance in everyday tasks

7. A patient diagnosed with insulin dependent diabetes mellitus is referred to occupational therapy for splinting. A primary area that must be assessed before prescribing a splint is:
   a. Edema
   b. Sensation
   c. Pain
   d. Fine motor manipulation

8. An OT is asked to administer a test to a child and compare the assessment results or scores to the sample population of children that have similar characteristics as this child. The BEST type of evaluation to administer would be:
   a. Criterion-referenced test
   b. Norm-referenced test
   c. Skilled observation
   d. Checklist

9. During an evaluation, the OT must determine a child's exact chronological age. The child was born on March 6, 2003 and the testing date is July 12, 2006. The child's chronological age is:
   a. 4 years, 6 months, 5 days
   b. 3 years, 2 months, 6 days
   c. 4 years, 5 months, 6 days
   d. 3 years, 4 months, 6 days

10. An OT has to calculate the corrected age for a child that was born prematurely. The child had a due date of September 20, 2005 and their birth date was June 12, 2005. The child was born 3 months, 8 days premature and is currently 1 year, 1 month, 25 days old. The therapist determines the corrected age is:
    a. 10 months, 17 days
    b. 12 months, 2 days
    c. 9 months, 8 days
    d. 7 months, 10 days

11. A 3-year-old child has been referred for early intervention. In the discussion about intervention with the family, the team should be sure to:
    a. Use lay terminology to describe the early intervention process
    b. Explain conditions in detailed technical and medical terms
    c. Discourage parents asking questions
    d. Ignore parents' feedback and ideas on intervention

12. A 6-year-old is interested in learning to roller skate. However, after the initial few minutes of practice the child does not continue with it and appears to lack the will to follow up what was started. This behavior is typical of Erik Eriksson's psychosocial development stage that deals with:
    a. Basic trust versus mistrust stage
    b. Autonomy versus doubt and shame stage
    c. Self-identity versus role diffusion stage
    d. Security versus instability

13. Which one of the four components of the adaptation process pertains to reception of sensory stimuli from internal and external environments?
    a. Assimilation
    b. Accommodation
    c. Association
    d. Differentiation

14. A 4-year-old has been diagnosed with mental retardation. A characteristic that is likely to occur with impaired intellectual ability is:
    a. Acceptable social skills
    b. Impairment of occupational performance areas
    c. Development of bizarre attachment to unusual objects
    d. Poor eye contact

15. A 3-year-old has accidentally ingested lead while playing near ceramic tiles that the family bought to renovate their house. A system that an OT working in pediatric acute care would note to be affected by lead poisoning would be:
    a. Vocal
    b. Circulatory
    c. Digestive
    d. Cardiac

16. A child with cerebral palsy shows significant impairment in the function of the lower extremities with mild involvement of the upper extremities. The classification of cerebral palsy for this child would be:
    a. Hemiplegia
    b. Tetraplegia
    c. Choreoathetosis
    d. Diplegia

17. A 7-year-old child is diagnosed with attention deficit hyperactivity disorder (ADHD). An etiology for ADHD would be:
    a. Environmental factors
    b. Visual and auditory stimulation
    c. Food allergies and food additives
    d. Neurochemical imbalances

18. A 5-year-old child has been diagnosed with a pervasive disorder that affects both the neurologic and motor behavioral functions. The diagnosis that MOST closely relates to the child's condition is:
    a. Respiratory distress syndrome
    b. Tourette's syndrome
    c. Asperger's syndrome
    d. Learning disabilities

19. A 5-year-old child with Down syndrome shows significant loss of weight, high fever, and paleness, and is diagnosed with acute lymphoid leukemia. In which of the following phases of leukemia will he be administered chemotherapy to treat small deposits of cells that remain after remission?
    a. Phase I—Induction therapy
    b. Phase II—Central nervous system prophylaxis
    c. Phase III—Intensification and consolidation
    d. Phase IV—Maintenance or continuation therapy

20. A 5-year-old child presents with difficulty climbing stairs, rising from a sitting or lying position, and demonstrates progressive fatigue caused by muscle weakness. The OT might suspect a problem with:
    a. Duchenne's muscular dystrophy

    b. Limb-girdle muscular dystrophy

    c. Facioscapulohumeral muscular dystrophy

    d. A congenital muscular dystrophy

21. The behavioral characteristics of autism, a pervasive developmental disorder (PDD), can be classified into four subclusters of disturbances. Of these disturbances, which is MOST closely related to prognosis?

    a. Disturbances in communication

    b. Disturbances in behaviors

    c. Disturbances in social interactions

    d. Disturbances of sensory and perceptual processing

22. A 3-year-old child is diagnosed with cerebral palsy and failure to thrive, and reportedly has difficulty with drooling, chewing, and swallowing. The OT should address:

    a. Oral motor deficits

    b. Motor sensory deficits

    c. Self-feeding

    d. Vestibular input

23. A kindergarten teacher observed that a 5-year-old child does not participate in play with other children and avoids movement activities on the playground. A screening test you would recommend for this child to determine if there is a need for a more comprehensive examination is:

    a. Ages & Stages Questionnaires

    b. The First STEP

    c. Short Sensory Profile

    d. Denver Developmental Screening Test-II (Denver-II)

24. A scenario in which an OT would use the School Function Assessment examination is:

    a. To measure the student's schoolwork task performance in the classroom and provide information for effective programs and consultation in the school setting

    b. To assess what the child "did do" and what the child "could do" to help determine the effect of the child's physical disability on engagement in everyday occupations

    c. For screening children to determine whether they warrant further, more comprehensive evaluation

    d. To measure children's ability to participate in the academic and social aspects of the school environment

25. An occupational therapy assistant (OTA) works with an OT in an early intervention program at a local school. The

portion of the evaluation that the OT can assign the OTA to perform is:

a. Selecting evaluation methods and measures
b. Interpreting and analyzing assessment data
c. Administering some of the assessments
d. Documenting some of the goals

26. A 3-year-old child has demonstrated delayed reflexes and locomotor skills and cannot grasp objects properly. The child trembles while walking and can't maintain balance. The therapist working with the child needs to obtain T scores and Z scores along with Developmental Motor Quotient scores. A test that would allow a therapist to obtain scores is:

a. Bayley Scales of Infant Development-II (BDSI-II)
b. Peabody Developmental Motor Scales-2 (PDMS-2)
c. Bruininks-Oseretsky Test of Motor Proficiency (BOTMP)
d. Pediatric Evaluation of Disability Inventory (PEDI)

27. A 5-month-old infant shows righting reactions of lifting its head when in the supine position. When the child is pulled to a sitting position, the child can maintain head alignment with the body without the initial head lag. The child's righting reaction is:

a. Neck on body reaction
b. Landau reaction
c. Body on head reaction
d. Flexion reaction

28. A child loses its balance and falls down whenever it tries to catch a ball thrown in its direction; otherwise the child can sit, stand, and walk well. The OT would determine that the child has a problem with:

a. Development of higher-level balance skills
b. Protective reactions
c. Anticipatory postural control
d. Labyrinthine head righting

29. A 4-year-old child is being assessed for possible vestibular disorder. In which of the following evaluation areas would the child face difficulties maintaining stance?

a. Eyes closed, stable platform
b. Eyes open, swayed-reference platform
c. Eyes closed, swayed-reference platform
d. Eyes open stable platform

30. The MOST complex skill that a 2-and-a-½ year-old child can demonstrate on the Peabody Developmental Motor Scales is:
    a. Snipping paper
    b. Cutting across a 6-inch piece of paper
    c. Cutting a circle
    d. Cutting a square

31. A 3-year-old child spends much time seated on the floor. The child supports this position by placing their left hand on the floor and cannot sit without the support. The child also demonstrates poor skills with its left hand. The general motor area that will MOST likely need attention first to help improve hand skills is:
    a. Inadequate isolation of movements
    b. Poorly graded movement
    c. Limitations in trunk movement and control
    d. Disorder in bilateral integration of movements

32. MOST infants first hold objects between the thumb and radial fingers at approximately:
    a. 4–5 months
    b. 6–7 months
    c. 8–9 months
    d. 10–11 months

33. A grasp that is often used to control tools or other objects is:
    a. Hook grasp
    b. Power grasp
    c. Lateral pinch
    d. Tip pinch

34. The MOST important information that an OT gains from assessing a child's ball throwing skills is the child's:
    a. Use of thumb opposition
    b. Voluntary release of the ball
    c. Sequence and timing of arm movements
    d. Accuracy in hitting a target area

35. The biomechanical frame of reference is MOST likely to be used in assessing and intervening for hand skills problems in children with:
    a. Motor planning difficulties
    b. Limitations in range of motion (ROM), strength, or endurance
    c. Tactile and/or proprioceptive sensory problems
    d. Postural tone and coordination problems

36. A problem that limits in-hand manipulation is:
    a. Limited finger isolation and control
    b. Inability to hold more than one object in the hand at the same time
    c. An inability to maintain long sitting
    d. Difficulty combining wrist extension with finger extension

37. A 4-year-old child avoids wearing clothes with waistbands, as well as socks and shoes, and also avoids having their hair combed. Dressing is a very difficult process each day. The OT would suspect that this behavior is caused by:
    a. Normal age appropriate behavior
    b. Avoidance of the sensation caused by elastic materials
    c. Sensory registration difficulty
    d. Sensory modulation difficulty

38. A 6-year-old child has an inability to discriminate vestibular proprioceptive stimuli. A function that would cause difficulties is:
    a. Judging the space between objects
    b. Perceiving form and space and relationships among objects
    c. Perceiving depth, distance, and location of boundaries
    d. Judging the correct force to use with people or objects

39. A sign of sensory integrative disorder is:
    a. Oversensitivity to touch, movement, sights, or sounds
    b. Inattentive impulsive behavior
    c. More active when compared to other children
    d. Impulsive behavior

40. The developmental stage that allows for discrimination and localization of tactile sensations to become more precise, and allows refinement of fine motor skills like grasping a pencil or manipulating Play Doh is:
    a. First 6 months
    b. Second 6 months
    c. 1–2 years
    d. 3–7 years

41. A child with mild spastic diplegia usually displays:
    a. Tactile defensiveness
    b. Gravitational insecurity
    c. Postural insecurity
    d. Overresponsiveness

42. A tendency to generate responses that are appropriately graded in
     relation to incoming sensory stimuli, rather than underreacting or
     overreacting to them, is called:
     a. Sensory registration
     b. Sensory modulation
     c. Sensation seeking
     d. Sensory discrimination

43. A condition that can cause double vision or mental suppression of
     one of the images that affect the development of visual perception is:
     a. Strabismus
     b. Phoria
     c. Myopia
     d. Astigmatism

44. A 10-year-old child is in the third grade. The child's parents are
     worried about the recent poor performance in math. The child's grades
     show that the child is age-appropriate in reading and writing, and that
     the child can perform simple subtraction and addition problems, but
     the child faces difficulty in solving problems that involve multiple steps
     or columns. This information should clue the OT to screen for:
     a. Visual-formation problems
     b. Visual-discrimination problems
     c. Object (form) problems
     d. Visual-spatial problems

45. An 8-month-old infant is not able to orient the hand properly for
     grasping before reaching and does not have any sensory deficits.
     The OT should assess:
     a. Depth perception
     b. Visual tracking
     c. Visual memory
     d. Visual attention

46. An 8-year-old tries to avoid reading lessons, is restless in the classroom,
     and when admonished complains of tired eyes. When made to read,
     the child often makes mistakes, such as reading "was" for "saw,"
     and makes errors in copying from the blackboard and exhibits poor
     spelling. The probable cause is:
     a. Impairment of topographic orientation
     b. Spatial vision problem
     c. Impairment of figure ground distinction
     d. Visual discrimination problems

47. A 9-year-old child has difficulty in focusing on tasks in school and is often not able to screen out unnecessary information. The child gets distracted by unrelated data and fails to obtain specific information necessary for the task. The OT should assess the child for difficulties with:
    a. Visual scanning
    b. Visual memory
    c. Selective attention
    d. Alertness

48. The MOST effective input channel for elementary school children to learn is:
    a. Auditory
    b. Visual
    c. Tactile
    d. Kinesthetic

49. A 2-year-old is reported by a patent as being shy and passive. The child does not show much enthusiasm for doing new things, playing with children, interacting with family, or going to new places. As the OT, the FIRST step would be to identify the child's temperament style before beginning to plan your intervention strategy. The temperament style that BEST describes this child is:
    a. Easy child
    b. Slow to warm up child
    c. Difficult child
    d. Forward child

50. A 6-year-old first grader is referred to occupational therapy by a teacher. The teacher observes that the child does not interact in the classroom and is extremely quiet. The child is typically sad and lacks enthusiasm for activities that classmates enjoy, and wants to take naps at recess. When presented with new challenges the child is sometimes tearful and makes self-deprecating remarks. The mental health diagnosis that the behavior MOST closely resembles is:
    a. Mood disorder
    b. Anxiety disorder
    c. Bipolar disorder
    d. PDD

51. A 7-year-old child is being evaluated by an OT for learning disabilities. The therapist observed that the child acts before thinking, often forgets things, and sometimes leaves schoolwork unfinished. When engaged in an activity the child continuously tries to redirect. The diagnosis that BEST describes the behavior is:
    a. Obsessive compulsive disorder
    b. ADHD
    c. PDD
    d. Childhood conduct disorder

52. A patient with a radial nerve injury is re-evaluated by the OT to assess the amount of sensory return as the nerve regenerates. The process for testing sensory return should include application of the stimulus:
    a. From proximal to distal on the anterior forearm, first, second, and third digits
    b. In random order to the anterior forearm, first, second, and third digits
    c. To the medial aspect of the forearm and digits
    d. In random order to the posterior lateral aspect of the forearm, and first three digits

53. A 40-year-old patient with a 3-week-old wrist fracture is receiving outpatient therapy focused on early mobilization. The OT should FIRST:
    a. Determine the patient's tolerance for pain
    b. View the radiographs to determine the amount of healing that has taken place
    c. Begin isometric exercise for strengthening
    d. Teach self-ranging and tendon gliding techniques

54. An OT must evaluate a patient who recently had a heart attack. What critical reasoning approach should be followed to establish the occupational profile?
    a. Narrative reasoning
    b. Pragmatic reasoning
    c. Scientific reasoning
    d. Ethical reasoning

55. To give an up-to-date report at the medical team meeting, the OT must report on the progress of the patient. The most up-to-date information should be obtained by performing a(n):
    a. Discharge summary/review of outcomes
    b. Occupational profile
    c. Initial evaluation
    d. Intervention review

56. When evaluating a client's shoulder's ROM, the therapist asks the client to move the upper extremity through the available active range of motion. The client was able to move the extremity through approximately half of its range, but required assistance to complete the full arc of motion. The OT would document that the muscle strength in this extremity is:
    a. Fair minus
    b. Good minus
    c. Fair
    d. Very poor

57. The OT needs to develop the occupational profile of a deaf client. The MOST appropriate assessment method to use would be:
    a. Interview a family member
    b. Provide a standardized test to the individual
    c. Do a home visit to observe the person in action
    d. Present a written inventory that the person can respond to

58. An 8-year-old child with a history of problems related to developmental dyspraxia has transferred to a new pediatric clinic. The OT at this facility would need to access the:
    a. Response to tactile stimulation
    b. Ability to initiate and complete a new activity
    c. Muscle strength and ROM
    d. Ability to recall numbers and letters

59. A patient recently experienced a nerve compress that caused the right dominant hand to be limp. Client factors affected are both sensory and motor, including no active wrist extension or forearm supination. Based on this scenario, the OT should assess:
    a. Motor and sensory problems affecting the posterior arm and fingers
    b. Sensory problems and edema of the involved extremity
    c. Paresthesia of the anterior aspect of the arm and fingers
    d. Motor and sensory problems associated with anterior arm and fingers

60. A patient with C6 tetraplegia is referred to an inpatient rehabilitation unit. The occupational therapy intervention plan should highlight the asset that:
    a. Normal bowel and bladder control are present
    b. Trunk stability is present
    c. There are no cognitive losses
    d. Motor control of the upper extremities is intact

61. A football athlete with an incomplete C7 spinal cord injury seeks the OT's opinion about the ability to live independently. The BEST response from the OT would be:

a. "You will be able to live independently with modifications such as adapted devices for activities of daily living (ADLs), a wheelchair, and sliding board."
b. "You can live along most of the time, but will require a caregiver for such tasks as driving, cooking, and ADLs."
c. "Persons with this level of spinal cord lesion will require an attendant."
d. "Persons with this level of injury can live independently with a manual wheelchair for mobility."

62. A patient with diabetes is employed as a bricklayer. The patient has recently developed a neuropathy leading to impaired sensation in the upper extremities. In regards to work, the OT needs to caution the patient to examine their hand frequently for:
a. Swelling and dryness
b. Bruising and redness
c. Dryness and erythema
d. Excessive perspiration

63. An individual who recently received radiation in the area of the head and neck drools, pockets food, and coughs. The OT should:
a. Recommend increasing liquid and a cough suppressant
b. Recommend a feeding tube
c. Provide intervention for dysphasia
d. Advise that these are common radiation reactions, which will disappear over time

64. A third-grade student who receives special education services has been hitting other children on the playground. The interdisciplinary team serving this student meets to develop an IEP. The FIRST step the team should follow from the activities list below is:
a. Make a decision and develop a plan for achieving the solution
b. Develop a comprehensive objective description of the problem
c. Get input from the other children that were recipient of the problem behaviors
d. Identify as many strategies as possible to reduce barriers and increase supports

65. The OT administered a norm-referenced test to a client who exhibited performance deficits with fine motor coordination. When scoring the test, the OT should:
a. Compare the patient's performance to the average score of a similar population
b. Compare the patient's performance to a defined list of skills
c. Compare the patient's performance to a specific objectives and normal function
d. Rate the patient's performance based on a progressive scale

66. A patient with rotator cuff repair surgery to the left nondominant shoulder 3 days ago is referred to occupational therapy for an evaluation. An assessment that might be contraindicated is:
    a. Sensory testing
    b. ROM testing
    c. Manual muscle testing
    d. Self-care assessment

67. A client with a shoulder impingement is referred to occupational therapy for skilled instructions in dressing. A dressing technique that would have a tendency to cause symptoms to increase is:
    a. Donning and doffing socks and shoes
    b. Pulling pants up to waist
    c. Putting on a shirt with buttons down the front
    d. Putting on an overhead garment

68. A client with a nerve resection is being evaluated for sensory return. The OT can BEST assess the client by:
    a. Tapping over the nerve to elicit feelings distal to the suture site
    b. Performing a manual muscle test of individual muscles
    c. Using test tubes filled with hot and cold water to distinguish differences in temperature
    d. Occluding vision and asking client to identify areas touched with a cotton ball

69. The OT is interested in determining the degree of sensory discrimination present in the fingertips of a patient with scleroderma. The BEST assessment to use is the:
    a. Fingertip wrinkling test
    b. Monofilament test
    c. Distinguishing between light and deep touch
    d. Test for stereognosis

70. A 65-year-old patient who sustained a myocardial infarction 1 week prior has been referred to cardiac rehabilitation. To determine the functional capacity, the OT should initially assess:
    a. Caregiver's ability to handle the patient at home
    b. Resumption of sexual activity with spouse
    c. Endurance for grooming, hygiene, dressing, and eating
    d. Ability to return to work on a part-time basis

71. A patient with an upper motor neuron spinal cord lesion at C6 began receiving occupational therapy 2 weeks after the injury. During the third week, the therapist notices an increase in spasticity. The therapist should:
    a. Conclude that symptoms are typical after spinal shock
    b. Conclude that the patient maybe in respiratory distress

    c. Suspect that a contracture is developing

    d. Look for signs of autonomic dysreflexia

72. A patient with diabetes mellitus also has complications of peripheral neuropathy. During the evaluation, the OT discovers that there are additional tactile processing issues. Further assessment should focus on:

    a. Visual deficits

    b. Fatigue and endurance

    c. Fine and gross coordination

    d. Reflexes

73. A patient with a diagnosis of lung cancer is referred to home health occupational therapy. The patient was forced to retire because of the illness and the OT would like to assess the patient's perception and satisfaction with the present level of occupational performance. The BEST type of assessment to use is:

    a. An interest checklist

    b. A standardized questionnaire

    c. A functional motion assessment

    d. A semi-structured interview

74. A 45-year-old with thoracic outlet syndrome has been in a work rehabilitation program for 3 weeks and is about to transition to part-time work at the local glass plant, the client's current place of employment. Before making the transition, an assessment of the client's ability to successfully perform their job duties is needed. The BEST approach for the OT to use to gather this data is through:

    a. Skilled observations

    b. Norm-referenced measurements

    c. Informal measures such as a checklist

    d. Standardized assessments

75. An 8-month-old preterm infant has obvious motor delays. The type of assessment that would enable the pediatric OT to determine the degree of the infant's delay is:

    a. Skilled observations

    b. Criterion referenced

    c. Interview with parents

    d. Ecological measures

76. The OT discovers that a patient cannot extend the elbow when positioned for manual muscle testing against gravity. In adjusting for the effects of gravity, the OT should position the patient:

    a. In sitting with humerus and elbow flexed and supported to 90 degrees

    b. In side lying with arm that being tested raised to shoulder level

    c. In supine with humerus and elbow flexed to 90 degrees

    d. In prone with arm abducted to 90 degrees

77. The OT is requested to evaluate a mechanic's ability to locate and use small tools. The MOST appropriate sensory assessment to use is:
    a. A monofilament test
    b. A test for stereognosis
    c. Two-point discrimination
    d. An asthesiometer

78. A common behavioral change in one-third to one-half of clients with a traumatic brain injury is:
    a. Inappropriate sexual behavior
    b. Increased initiation with tasks
    c. Posttraumatic agitation
    d. Bizarre verbalizations

79. The MOST valid and valuable information attained during a motor evaluation to determine the functional level of a client with hemiplegia and resultant upper extremity spasticity would be:
    a. Gross sensory evaluation
    b. Standard manual muscle test
    c. Active range of motion (AROM)
    d. Observation of self-care performance

80. While performing a grooming evaluation, a client is noted to smear toothpaste over their hands and face. The OT should assess the client for possible issues with:
    a. Ideational apraxia
    b. Ideomotor apraxia
    c. Spatial relations deficit
    d. Motor apraxia

81. An OT is evaluating the degree of spasticity present in a client's right upper extremity. There is no active movement, but the therapist determines that there is resistance to passive movement; however, full ROM can be achieved. The degree of spasticity describe is generally classified as:
    a. Mild
    b. Moderate
    c. Severe
    d. Fluctuating

82. When evaluating a client you use a cross out sheet and a balloon activity. You are MOST concerned with:
    a. Visual scanning
    b. Visual acuity
    c. Ocular control
    d. Visual perception

83. A 65-year-old client had a right stroke in the nondominant hemisphere of the parietal lobe. During an ADL evaluation, the client dresses the unaffected limb but not the affected limb. This is an indication of:
    a. Visual field cut
    b. Ideomotor apraxia
    c. Unilateral body neglect
    d. Ideational apraxia

84. An OT asks a patient to demonstrate how to brush the teeth; the patient then picks up the toothbrush by the bristles with a tip-to-tip pinch. This is caused by:
    a. Difficulty with visual figure-ground
    b. Ideomotor apraxia
    c. Ideational apraxia
    d. Semantic memory loss

85. Hemianopsia is a loss of visual field secondary to a stroke. The MOST probable visual loss for a right cerebrovascular accident (CVA) would be:
    a. Temporal side of the right eye and the nasal side of the left eye
    b. Nasal side of the left eye and the nasal side of the right eye
    c. Nasal side of right eye and temporal side of left eye
    d. Nasal and temporal sides of the left eye only

86. Some children tend to seek out large quantities of intense sensory stimulation. This "sensory seeking" behavior is thought to be related to a sensory system that is:
    a. Hyporesponsive
    b. Hyperresponsive
    c. Defensive
    d. High registering

87. A child has difficulty recognizing letters in different styles of print or in making the transition from printed to cursive letters. The child has a visual discrimination problem of:
    a. Form constancy
    b. Spatial vision
    c. Figure ground perception
    d. Binocular fusion

88. An OT is working with a child that is suspected of having difficulties with visual perceptual skill. Developmentally, the FIRST visual component that needs to be assessed is:
    a. Pattern recognition
    b. Scanning skills
    c. Visual attention
    d. Oculomotor control

89. An elementary student has been referred to you for a comprehensive handwriting assessment. Your FIRST priority would be:
    a. Administering a standardized visual perceptual test
    b. Evaluating the student's actual performance in handwriting
    c. Assessing the student's performance in the context of the classroom
    d. Interviewing the child's parents, teachers, and other team members

90. While doing a worksite assessment in the hospital business office, an OT found several employees complaining of neck and shoulder pain. It was determined that making a simple change in the set-up of the computer stations could reduce symptoms. The change to the computer monitor that would MOST affect neck and shoulder discomfort is:
    a. Lower the monitor to the desk surface
    b. Move the computer monitor closer to the employee's face
    c. Tilt monitor forward
    d. Put a non-glare screen on the monitor

91. The OT is advising a patient who is returning to work after being treated for a nerve compression at the elbow on positioning. The OT should include in the list of instructions that it is important to avoid:
    a. Postures that involve elbow flexion
    b. Postures that involve elbow extension
    c. Direct pressure to the affected area
    d. Reaching downward

92. An OT developed neck and shoulder pain after just 20 minutes of using a laptop computer at home but not after 1 hour of using the desktop computer at work. The MOST likely reason for this is:
    a. Small mouse in center of keyboard
    b. Small keyboard with no wrist rest
    c. Smaller screen size
    d. Decreased contrast on screen

93. The optimal workspace for a worker seated at a table is:
    a. 12 inches to either side of midline and 12 inches in front of the worker

b. Approximately 1 hand span width directly in front of the worker
c. 180 degree arc from left side of table to right side of table
d. Any area that can be reached with shoulders at 15 degrees adduction and 0 degrees flexion

94. An OT is treating a teacher who was injured in a motor vehicle accident and is now in a wheelchair. The school has requested an ergonomic assessment to modify the teacher's classroom. The OT recommends lowering the chalkboard. Without knowing the teacher's height, the highest height for the top of the chalkboard that the OT would recommend is:
   a. 36 inches
   b. 42 inches
   c. 48 inches
   d. 52 inches

95. An OT is doing a home assessment for a client who will be going home in a wheelchair. The patient is a gourmet cook and wants to put an island in the kitchen for food preparation. The sink is on one wall, with the refrigerator on the wall to the left and the stove/oven on the wall to the right. The client will need to be able to turn all the way around in the wheelchair to access everything. The minimum space required is:
   a. 40-inch square
   b. 55-inch square
   c. 62-inch square
   d. 74-inch square

96. A patient recently diagnosed with a left CVA presents with symptoms of bilateral upper extremity tremors, edema in the right fingers, dorsum of the hand, and enlarged DIP joints. However, good return of function is noted proximal to the wrist. In the early phase of rehabilitation, the OT should focus on splinting to:
   a. Correct contractures
   b. Prevent secondary complications
   c. Decrease pain
   d. Substitute for sensorimotor function

97. A 2-year-old client with delayed motor skills shifts his weight onto one leg and steps to the side with the other in a movement pattern described as:
   a. Dancing
   b. Creeping
   c. Cruising
   d. Crawling

98. The parents of a 7-year-old describe their child as having severe difficulty in communicating and interacting with others. On observation, the OT noticed repetitive and ritualistic behaviors. These behaviors are MOST likely associated with:
    a. Childhood conduct disorder
    b. ADHD
    c. Obsessive-compulsive disorder
    d. PDD

99. A 6-year-old child presents with increased tone of the right upper and lower extremities, including flexion contractures of the elbow and wrist and the thumb adducted in a fisted hand. The child also has mild flexion contracture of the right knee and walks on the toes. The OT would plan assessments and interventions appropriate for:
    a. Spastic diplegia
    b. Flaccid paraplegia
    c. Spastic hemiplegia
    d. Flaccid monoplegia

100. A child uses a wide-base of support when walking because of instability and poor weight shifting. This is characteristic of:
    a. Mental retardation
    b. Scoliosis
    c. Juvenile rheumatoid arthritis
    d. Ataxic cerebral palsy

101. A preschool child has been referred to occupational therapy for a screening. The OT's next step is to:
    a. Observe the child's developmental behaviors
    b. Establish a treatment plan
    c. Gather information from the teachers and parents
    d. Determine the need for further evaluation

102. The OT would administer a test of visual-motor integration to a child who MOST likely has difficulty with:
    a. Copying letters
    b. Putting puzzles together
    c. Selecting geometric shapes that are the same
    d. Finding a figure embedded in a beach scene

103. An 8-month-old infant assumes a quadruped position and then rocks back and forth; this behavior indicates:
    a. Repetitive behaviors
    b. Normal development
    c. Fluctuating muscle tone
    d. Being stuck in a movement pattern

104. An elementary school conducted a "spine screening"; two students were noted to have an exaggerated curvature of the thoracic spine. This is characteristic of:
    a. Lordosis
    b. Kyphosis
    c. Lumbardosis
    d. Pulmonary infusion

105. In order for a person to receive services available for developmental disability, he or she must meet the criteria of a condition that has:
    a. Early onset, but brief manifestation in limited functioning
    b. Onset of the condition before the age of 22
    c. Physical dysfunctions with an onset after age 7
    d. Onset prior to preschool years

106. Among children who are autistic, the MOST significant area of impairment tends to be:
    a. Social
    b. Cognitive
    c. Self-care
    d. Motor

107. An OT assessing movement determines that a child has oscillating vision. An area for further assessment might be:
    a. Eye–hand coordination
    b. Equilibrium
    c. Muscle tone
    d. Drawing ability

108. A psychosocial reaction of an elderly client who experiences difficulty understanding normal speech sounds might be:
    a. Decreased physical reactions
    b. Decreased paranoid tendencies
    c. Increased social activities
    d. Increased paranoid tendencies

109. An OT might encourage a 70-year-old client to use a slower gait:
    a. So that the client can conserve energy to prevent muscle fatigue
    b. Because walking at a speed consistent with the client's age is most appropriate
    c. So that the client can adjust better to the physical activity
    d. To prevent overexerting the heart and other bodily systems

110. An elderly client with no visual deficits exhibits difficulty with balance and also reports a tendency to occasionally fall. The OT should assess:
    a. Labyrinthine righting reflexes
    b. Tactile discrimination
    c. Vestibular function
    d. Visual memory

111. During a home health visit, the OT observed several items that require modification in the home of an elderly patient. In terms of priority, the environmental hazard that needs the MOST immediate attention is:
    a. The cracked toilet seat
    b. A malfunctioning thermostat
    c. A throw rug
    d. A cluttered kitchen

112. As a person ages, the OT must be concerned about the individual's capabilities along a continuum of mental or cognitive functioning, also known as:
    a. Biological age
    b. Chronological age
    c. Social age
    d. Psychological age

113. An elderly client is observed by an OT as having an unsteady gait, and the client has to hold onto the wall when coming in and out of the bathroom. The OT should assess the patient for:
    a. Visual deficits
    b. Postural control
    c. A possible wheelchair or walker
    d. Apraxia

114. An older person with functional impairments and poor physiological reserve who has difficulty living independently is known as the:
    a. Elderly
    b. Frail elderly
    c. Vulnerable aged
    d. Aged adult

115. Family structures change through births, deaths, and marriages. The social context that BEST illustrates this is:
    a. Family structures are static.
    b. Families are ruled by tradition.
    c. Family housing is changed periodically.
    d. Family structures are dynamic.

116. An OT is assessing sensation in a 75-year-old patient. The results show decreased light touch and normal protective sensation. The therapist should document that:
    a. Sensation is significantly impaired
    b. Sensation is appropriate for age
    c. Further testing is needed
    d. Stereognosis should be tested

117. A client's loss of ROM, grip strength, and sensation caused by a work-related injury would be documented by the OT as a(n):
    a. Handicap
    b. Disability
    c. Dysfunction
    d. Impairment

118. An OT would expect a patient that presents with performance deficits caused by issues related to visual processing to demonstrate difficulties with:
    a. Tracking
    b. Attending to objects
    c. Focusing on multiple objects
    d. Discrimination between objects

119. The Individuals with Disabilities Education Act (IDEA) of 1990 mandates the inclusion of specific transition services in a student's IEP when the student reaches 16 years of age. The MOST appropriate contribution to the transition process by occupational therapy would be evaluation of the student's:
    a. Mobility and gait-related skills
    b. Communication and process skills
    c. Job-related interests and abilities to facilitate worker–job match
    d. Participation in the classroom to facilitate skills

120. An OT, consulting with a business, has been asked to develop employment pre-placement screening for the employees. According the American with Disabilities Act of 1990 (ADA; Public Law 101-336), the employer cannot ask certain information during the employment preplacement screening. The OT must advise the employer of ADA compliance issues. The type of information the employer could request during the preplacement screening is:
    a. Can the applicant meet the physical demands of the job?
    b. What medical condition(s) does the applicant have?
    c. What type of disability does the applicant have?
    d. What medications does the applicant currently take?

121. A client with a diagnosis of C6 cervical disc herniation secondary to forceful cervical flexion injury at work is seen in an outpatient rehabilitation clinic. On examination by the OT, the client complains of pain, weakness, and paresthesia in their right upper extremity. The MOST likely cause of the patient's right upper extremity symptoms is:
    a. Double crush syndrome
    b. Cervical radiculopathy
    c. Carpal tunnel syndrome
    d. Thoracic outlet syndrome

122. An upper-extremity musculoskeletal disorder that would be considered a work-related condition is:
    a. Primary thumb carpal–metacarpal osteoarthritis
    b. Cervical stenosis
    c. Lateral epicondylitis
    d. Dupuytren's contracture

123. The OT is evaluating a client with a "suspected" work-related musculoskeletal disorder. During an occupational interview with the client, the OT determines that the client is exposed to multiple risk factors. Which of the following is considered a work-related risk factor for developing a musculoskeletal disorder?
    a. Sedentary lifestyle
    b. Obesity
    c. Awkward postures
    d. Diabetes

124. Prior to discharge, the OT needs to determine how efficient a patient is when performing morning ADLs. The BEST measure to use is to assess:
    a. The amount of time it takes to complete the self-care tasks
    b. The complexity of the tasks that need to be done during the morning
    c. If pain is present when performing the morning self-care routine
    d. The number of times adapted equipment is used during the morning routine

125. A client on temporary leave from work at a factory that manufactures dental supplies is referred to an occupational rehabilitation program for therapy and work reconditioning. The OT gathers data on the organization, its senior level management, and demographic of the employees. Contextually, the OT is addressing:
    a. The physical work environment

b. The social work environment
c. The political and cultural work environment
d. The personal and temporal work environment

126. A 54-year-old client sustained a work-related lateral epicondylitis in the right dominant upper extremity. The OT assesses the work environment, including the client's ability to use a screwdriver frequently to assemble circuit boards. According to the *OT Practice Framework*, the component that is being assessed in this manner is the client's:
a. Body function and body structure
b. Activity demands
c. Social routines and habits
d. Sequencing and timing skills

127. The OT conducts a worksite visit and assesses an injured client's workstation. The information gathered by the OT will be used to first:
a. Develop an occupational profile
b. Analyze occupational performance
c. Develop an intervention plan
d. Implement an intervention plan

128. The occupational therapy supervisor of an occupational rehabilitation program is contacted by a case manager regarding the program's functional capacity evaluation (FCE) services. A workers' compensation case manager wanted to know more about the utility of FCEs for their clients. The OT should list all of the following as possible roles of FCEs in occupational rehabilitation EXCEPT:
a. To determine if a work-related impairment exists
b. To establish a rehabilitation treatment plan for an injured worker
c. To determine at what level a return to work would be appropriate
d. To determine employability of workers with impairments

129. The OT is required to perform an evaluation to determine the maximum amount of weight the client can lift, push, pull, and carry. According the *OT Practice Framework: Domain and Process,* the client's maximum capacity for lifting, pushing, pulling, and carrying is an assessment of:
a. Job performance
b. Employment capacity
c. Physicality
d. Strength and effort

130. During a mental health group exercise, the OT provides the participants with an activity that requires them to interact, share ideas, and provide directions to each other in order to make successful progress from one step to another. MOST likely the OT is facilitating:
    a. Information exchange
    b. Verbal and nonverbal communication
    c. Social play
    d. Physical interaction

131. An individual suspected of having a work-related de Quervain's condition is referred for an evaluation. The MOST appropriate provocative test for the OT to perform during the initial evaluation is:
    a. Phalen's
    b. Grind
    c. Cozens
    d. Finklestein's

132. The OT consultant interviews the human resource director and floor supervisor of a manufacturing plant. The OT learns that the company has been negatively affected by recent changes in statues set forth by the Occupational Safety and Health Administration (OSHA). According to the *OT Practice Framework: Domain and Process,* this information provides the OT with a better understanding of the organization's:
    a. Social context
    b. Virtual environment
    c. Physical context
    d. Cultural context

133. A 23-year-old client sustained a work-related carpal tunnel syndrome in their right dominant hand. Past medical history is unremarkable. The OT assessed the demands in the work environment, which indicated that the client was required to utilize a power sander frequently ($1/3$ to $2/3$ of the day) to sand unfinished wood furniture. The work-related risk factor the OT would MOST likely describe as the strongest contributor to the client's carpal tunnel syndrome is:
    a. Excessive vibration
    b. Forceful pinching
    c. Excessive finger movements
    d. Static upper extremity postures

134. A child who lacks the automatic ability to modulate auditory information is in a classroom full of children who are being instructed in a math lesson. While the teacher is reviewing how to subtract fractions, the child may:
    a. Cover their eyes to block visual input

b. Start rocking back and forth to increase vestibular input

c. Cover their ears to block out the teacher's voice

d. Get up and start dancing to music they hear off in the distance

135. An OT is working in the school system with a 7-year-old child who has severely impaired cognition and motor abilities. The child requires a great deal of assistance with feeding, toileting, and other basic self-care tasks. It is MOST likely that the OT will choose an assessment that measures:

a. Gross motor and fine motor skills

b. Visual motor integration skills

c. Achievement toward developmental milestones

d. A child's ability to participate in self-care, mobility, and social functions

136. An OT is working in an outpatient hand clinic with an 11-year-old child who has a diagnosis of juvenile rheumatoid arthritis. After completing an occupational profile, the OT decides that it would be beneficial to further assess the child's skills. The OT will MOST likely choose an assessment that measures:

a. Gross motor and fine motor skills

b. Visual motor integration skills

c. Achievement toward developmental milestones

d. Processing and communication stills

137. An OT is working with a child to develop age-appropriate hand skills. Before beginning the session, the OT makes sure that the treatment room is well lit so that the child will have the maximum advantage of using their visual skills. Vision is important for the development of hand skills because:

a. Vision provides motivation and feedback for motor movements.

b. Vision provides a child with a sense to determine if an object is heavy or light.

c. Vision and hand skill develop at the same rate.

d. The use of color vision attracts children to novel objects that they want to explore.

138. An OT is working with a child who demonstrates persistent primitive reflexes after a brain injury. The OT is working with the child to actively grasp and release blocks. The child is having difficulty releasing the blocks into a bin. This is MOST likely caused by the persistence of the:

a. Asymmetrical tonic neck reflex

b. Avoiding response

c. Traction response

d. Grasp reflex

139. The occupational therapy student (OTS) is trying to describe how a child's eyes look to the student's supervisor. The OTS notices that at times one of the child's eyes turns out ever so slightly and the child has reported double vision. The OT supervising the OTS explains that the child's history includes information indicating that the child's eyes are misaligned, causing a condition called:
    a. Myopia
    b. Esotropia
    c. Strabismus
    d. Amblyopia

140. An OT is interviewing a child's parent as part of an initial evaluation. Among other things, the child's parent mentions that the child often complains of being nauseated after riding on an escalator. The OT suspects that the child might have a sensory integrative dysfunction related to poor processing of:
    a. Tactile information
    b. Visual information
    c. Vestibular information
    d. Auditory information

141. An OT is providing early intervention services to an infant that was 13 weeks premature. The infant's parent reports that the child cries and tenses in an extension pattern when picked up and fed, or if the diaper is changed. However, the child tends to calm down and accepts a bottle readily when placed in the care seat. The OT should evaluate this child for:
    a. Sensory defensiveness
    b. Inadequate anticipatory behaviors
    c. Sensory registration difficulties
    d. Difficulty regulating postural mechanism

142. An OT is working as part of an acute rehabilitation team at a children's hospital. The OT is given an order to make static splints for a 14-year-old child who has just received a continuous intrathecal baclofen pump. It is MOST likely that this pump was put in place to reduce:
    a. Curvature of the spine
    b. Seizure activity
    c. Pressure in the brain caused by hydrocephalus
    d. Spasticity

143. An OT is taking a developmental history for a 3-year-old child. During the interview, the OT learns that the child experienced a breech delivery. The OT later observes the child and finds the arm in an awkward position with the shoulder adducted and internally

rotated, elbow extended, forearm pronated, and wrist flexed. This posture is characteristic of:
a. Atrophy of shoulder girdle muscles
b. Upper motor neuron lesion
c. Brachial plexus lesion
d. Spinal nerve injury

144. An OT is working with a 4-year-old on buttoning a series of three large buttons. The child is successful with unbuttoning and performing other tasks that require the same level of fine motor dexterity but continues to have difficulty buttoning. The OT may decide to further assess the child's:
a. Pinch strength
b. Perceptual abilities
c. Upper extremity strength
d. Sensory regulation skills

145. An OT is working with a fourth-grade student who has difficulty with handwriting. The child's work samples show that the child is unable to consistently write text within the writing guidelines. This is a problem with:
a. Letter formation
b. Alignment
c. Spacing
d. Near-point copying

146. An OT chooses to evaluate a child using the Sensory Profile developed by Dunn. The OT is hoping to gain information:
a. That links the child's sensory processing abilities with performance in typical ADLs
b. Related to the child's ability to balance and use bilaterally coordinated movements
c. That explains the child's difficulty with ideation, planning, and execution of motor sequences at home and at school
d. That informs treatment planning for concerns related to functional communication

147. An OT is working with a child with Down syndrome to put on a pair of pierced earrings. The child MOST likely has difficulty with this task because of:
a. A short hand
b. Delayed bone ossification
c. A lower set thumb
d. Hypotonia

148. A student with ADHD constantly looks up to the chalkboard while copying information. In addition to concerns related to maintaining attention, the student MOST likely has difficulty with:
    a. Visual discrimination
    b. Visual closure
    c. Visual memory
    d. Position in space

149. A child who is averse to vestibular input may experience the following reaction immediately after going down a playground slide:
    a. Dizziness and nausea
    b. Avoidance of touch
    c. Difficulty sequencing the actions needed to climb on the monkey bars without assistance
    d. Increased muscle tone throughout trunk

150. A child with sensory integration dysfunction who has difficulty with anticipatory projected movement sequences would also have difficulty:
    a. Organize movements to climb up the stairs
    b. Developing a motor plan to use scissors to cut out picture for a collage
    c. Using two hands together to fly a kite
    d. Catching a ball that is thrown

151. An OT working with a child receiving early intervention services and using the neuromaturational theory of development assumes that the child's rate of motor development is:
    a. Dependent on multiple variables
    b. Determined by the interaction between the child's individual systems and the child's context
    c. Dependent on low-level skills that are required as a foundation for higher-level skills
    d. Dependent on the caregiver's influence and the culture in which the child is being raised

152. A child with spastic diplegic cerebral palsy is referred for occupational therapy. MOST likely the child will present with functional deficits related to:
    a. Moderate involvement in all four extremities
    b. Involvement in upper and lower extremities on one side of the body
    c. Mild involvement in upper extremities and significant involvement in lower extremities
    d. Involvement in lower extremities only

153. An OT working in the school system is choosing an evaluation tool to use with a fourth-grade student who is having difficulty with handwriting. The OT would like to be able to compare the student's performance on this assessment to the performance of other students who have taken the same assessment. The OT would MOST likely choose a:
    a. Standardized assessment
    b. Criterion-referenced assessment
    c. Norm-referenced assessment
    d. Observation-based assessment

154. A 6-month-old child who was born at 30 weeks' gestation is being evaluated to determine eligibility for early intervention services. The child's adjusted age is approximately:
    a. 2 months
    b. 2.5 months
    c. 3 months
    d. 3.5 months

155. An OT is working with a child who presents with delayed in-hand manipulation skills. The OT is working with the child to develop simple rotation skills, which are necessary to unscrew a bottle top. The child will MOST likely also need this in-hand manipulation skill to:
    a. Pick up a small piece of cereal that is placed at midline to self-feed
    b. Move a key from the palm to the fingers to place in a lock
    c. Pick up a pencil that is placed horizontally with the writing end pointing toward the ulnar side of the child's preferred hand
    d. Move a coin from the finger pads to the finger tips to place inside of a bank

156. An OT is evaluating a 14-month-old child. According to typical development, the child should be able to:
    a. Jump up and down without external support
    b. Bend down to pick up a toy off the ground without external support
    c. Stand without external support
    d. Walk without external support

157. While working in a clinic, the OT concludes that a child has gravitational insecurity. According to the Sensory Integration theory, this issue is MOST significantly connected to the:
    a. Proprioceptive system
    b. Tactile system
    c. Auditory system
    d. Vestibular system

158. An OT is preparing to evaluate a child in the school systems and would like to use a top-down approach. It is likely that one of the first things that the OT will do as part of the assessment is choose an assessment that measures:
    a. How much the child participates at school
    b. The child's visual motor skills
    c. The child's fine motor strength
    d. The child's time on task

159. An OT is working with a 16-year-old student with a mental impairment who is interested in getting a part-time job. As part of therapy, the OT asks the student to complete a self-assessment that will yield information regarding the child's values and sense of volition. It is MOST likely that the OT is working within the theoretical framework of the:
    a. Acquisitional Learning theory
    b. Person Environment Occupation model
    c. Model of Human Occupation (MOHO)
    d. Canadian Occupational Performance model

160. A 9-month-old infant experiences some difficulties with spoon-feeding. While the OT is observing the caregiver feeding the infant, it is noted that the infant demonstrates a rhythmic in-and-out pattern of tongue movement. This movement pattern can BEST be described as tongue:
    a. Retraction
    b. Instability
    c. Tip elevation
    d. Thrust

161. During an interview with the caregiver of a 6-month-old, the OT is told that the infant is right-hand dominant. Based on this information, the OT concludes that:
    a. The child's development may be advanced
    b. The child's hand dominance may be indicative of central nervous system dysfunction
    c. The caregiver may only be presenting toys to the right of the child.
    d. The child sleeps in the prone position

162. A child is having difficulty catching a ball with two hands. The OT wishes to further evaluate the child's bilateral integration skills in the context of a functional activity. The OT will likely see if the child is successful when:
    a. Shifting weight on to one leg in preparation for kicking a ball with the opposite foot
    b. Swiping at a balloon with either hand
    c. Throwing a tennis ball at a target

    d.   Holding paper with one hand and using scissors to cut with the opposite hand

163. An OT is asked to assess a child's handwriting. During an observation, the OT notes that the child holds their pencil by resting it against the distal phalanx of the radial side of the middle finger while the pads of the thumb and index finger control it. This grip can best be described as:
    a.   Dynamic tripod grasp
    b.   Lateral tripod grasp
    c.   Modified tripod grasp
    d.   Quadripod grasp

164. Praxis, or motor planning, is comprised of three distinct components. They are:
    a.   Ideation, planning, and execution
    b.   Ideation, execution, and follow through
    c.   Ideation, planning, and sequencing
    d.   Ideation, problem solving, and preparing

165. According to the Sensory Integration theory, three senses are considered to have the most impact on a child's ability to process sensory information and produce an adaptive response. These senses are:
    a.   Auditory, tactile, and vestibular
    b.   Visual, vestibular, and proprioceptive
    c.   Visual, auditory, and olfactory
    d.   Vestibular, proprioceptive, and tactile

166. The parent of a child with Asperger's syndrome shares with the OT that when the child is playing at the park, the child often enjoys climbing on the monkey bars and jumping down. The parent reports that the child is regularly encouraged to play ball, go into the sandbox, and/or ride on the swings. However, the child usually refuses and continues to climb on to the top of the monkey bars and jump off. Based on this information, it MOST likely that the child is:
    a.   Avoiding playing with other children and interacting with his parent
    b.   Hyposenstive to tactile input
    c.   Seeking tactile input
    d.   Seeking vestibular and proprioceptive input

167. A 65-year-old client has sustained a mild left CVA. You are currently seeing the client on the inpatient rehabilitation unit. The client is independent with all self-care and basic ADLs. The client desires to go home and live alone. The BEST evaluation tool to use in this situation is:

a. Barthel Index
b. The Kohlman Evaluation of Living Skills
c. Functional Independence Measure
d. Functional Test for the Hemiparetic Upper Extremity

168. You are evaluating a 25-year-old client who has sustained a brain injury from a motor vehicle accident. During your motor evaluation of the elbow the client demonstrates nonvoluntary repetitive contractions of the biceps. This is described as:
a. Synergy
b. Clonus
c. Flaccidity
d. Spinal hypertonia

169. You are evaluating the motor control of a 65-year-old client who sustained a brain stem CVA 3 months ago. When performing the finger to nose test, the client reach seems to have:
a. Ataxia
b. Chorea
c. Ballism
d. Athetoid movement

170. The first step in a visual assessment of a 50-year-old patient who has sustained a brain injury would be:
a. Tracking
b. Visual field confrontation testing
c. Convergence testing
d. Visual history

171. You work in an acute care facility and have been asked to see a 70-year-old patient. While the patient is sitting, you observe that the client positions their left arm a flexed elbow and hand pulled to their body. You want to evaluate the client's tone the BEST evaluation for this is:
a. Ashworth
b. Wolf
c. Manual muscle test
d. Jebsen

172. You are seeing an 80-year-old client with a diagnosis of Parkinson's disease. Your motor evaluation reveals resistance throughout passive range of motion (PROM) of bilateral upper extremities with all speeds of movement. This would be BEST described as:
a. Hypertonus
b. Spasticity

    c. Rigidity

    d. Clonus

173. You are working on an inpatient rehabilitation unit and are assigned a 25-year-old client who has sustained a brain injury from a gunshot wound. As you enter the client's room, the client is eating breakfast. The client states that they are done eating breakfast, but you notice that only food on the right side of the tray has been eaten. Though a full evaluation of visual abilities is needed, you suspect that the client is dealing with which of the following:

    a. Left inattention

    b. Right field cut

    c. Decreased oculomotor control

    d. Diplopia

174. You are evaluating a 75-year-old client who has been diagnosed with a CVA. Your first visit is during a morning ADL routine. The client is currently sitting in a wheelchair at the sink and is requesting to brush their teeth. Several performance skills can be evaluated during this task. A behavior that would demonstrate a spatial relations deficit is:

    a. Forgetting to turn off the water

    b. Requiring verbal cues to put the toothbrush into their mouth

    c. Requiring verbal cues to put the toothpaste on the brush before brushing their teeth

    d. Requiring assistance for positioning the toothbrush under the faucet

175. The following performance skill deficit may be seen after a spinal cord injury:

    a. Aphasia

    b. Clonus

    c. Agnosia

    d. Apraxia

176. An OT is attempting to evaluate the reading ability of a patient who has sustained a right CVA with some difficulty. The patient reports that they typically use reading glasses but cannot locate them. Instead of ending the session, the OT could compensate by:

    a. Increasing print size

    b. Turning off the TV

    c. Reading the questions to the patient

    d. Writing words in red on a pink paper

177. A 19-year-old patient sustained a right CVA. Even though you are seated in a quiet environment the patient seems very slow in

answering your questions. From the patient's behavior you feel that the patient needs further assessment for:

a. Inattention
b. Receptive aphasia
c. Expressive aphasia
d. Delayed processing of information

178. A 55-year-old patient sees an OT for an evaluation of upper extremity function 1 week after Botox to the patient's finger flexors in the right upper extremity. The patient had a stroke 1 year ago and is continuing to work on increasing function. During your evaluation you find that you are unable to fully extend the wrist and the fingers. One of the goals you establish with the patient is to increase ROM in this area. The BEST way to achieve this goal is by:

a. AROM
b. PROM
c. Splinting to provide low load prolonged stretch
d. Stretching and weight bearing

179. You are evaluating a 67-year-old patient who had a stroke 3 weeks ago, and this is your fourth day of therapy in the patient's room. The patient has begun ambulating with hand hold assist during the last 2 days. On both visits while assisting the patient during ambulation to the bathroom, the patient is unable to find the bathoom located in the room. This would be an example of:

a. Lack of orientation
b. Topographical disorientation
c. Visual field cut
d. Homonymous hemianopsia

180. An OT must evaluate a patient who recently had a heart attack. A critical reasoning approach to follow to establish an occupational profile is:

a. Narrative reasoning
b. Pragmatic reasoning
c. Scientific reasoning
d. Ethical reasoning

181. A 9-year-old with anxiety has recently started taking a psychotropic medication. An OT is working with the child to improve handwriting and attention skills. The child has started complaining of dryness of the mouth and constipation. The BEST approach to address these symptoms would be:

a. Increase the fiber in the child's diet to improve the constipation and increase fluid intake for the dryness
b. Suggest an appointment with the child's primary care physician for a physical check up

    c. Suggest referring to the prescribing psychiatrist. These may be side effects of the drugs that the child is taking

    d. Suggest to the child's parents that the child begin an exercise regimen to increase bowel activity

182. An 8-year-old third-grader is generally well-behaved. The child's parents are very fastidious. The child is very particular about keeping their room and table tidy. While doing these tasks, the child restarts and repeats the process again and again. If the child is not allowed to continue the activity for as long as they want, they become anxious and begs to be allowed to finish. This behavior can BEST be described as:
    a. ADHD
    b. Bipolar disorder
    c. Obsessive-compulsive disorder
    d. Schizophrenia

183. Characteristics of PDD are:
    a. Normal sensory processing
    b. Restricted, repetitive patterns of behavior, interests, and activities
    c. Pervasive long-standing feelings of uneasiness
    d. Difficulty with selective or sustained attention to tasks

184. As an OT, it is important to know the basis of an infant's oral tactile defensiveness before planning an intervention program that could help resolve it. A possible cause of oral hypersensitivity would be:
    a. Procedures in the oropharyngeal area as a newborn
    b. Poor nutritional intake as an infant
    c. Low birth weight
    d. Respiratory problems from birth

185. A child should be able to go to the toilet independently but may still require some assistance with cleaning and clothing adjustment at:
    a. 1½ years
    b. 2½ years
    c. 3 years
    d. 4–5 years

186. A 3-year-old with autism has severe sensory integrative problems. A characteristic the child is likely to display would be:
    a. Stereotyped movements or types of play
    b. High play organization
    c. Limited and abnormal movement
    d. Engagement in social play with 2–3 people at a time

187. An OT has identified that a child exhibits certain features of creating letters that affect legibility, such as improper letterforms and poor leading in and leading out of letters. A feature that would also significantly affect legibility would be:
    a. Incomplete closure of letters
    b. Insufficient orientation of letters on the baseline
    c. Poor orientation of letters on line
    d. Inconsistency of slant

188. A typically developing 5½-month-old infant is able to roll easily from prone to supine positions and vice versa. Assuming that locomotion skills continue to develop at an average rate, the child would reach this mobility milestone at 9 months:
    a. Creeping and moving from sitting to quadruped and back
    b. Pivoting in the prone position
    c. Standing and cruising along furniture
    d. Ambulating upright and independently

189. A 7-year-old needs augmentative mobility. The OT has identified the child as a "marginal ambulatory." The condition that this describes is:
    a. A progressive neuromuscular disorder
    b. Cerebral palsy with less involvement
    c. Osteogenesis imperfecta
    d. Spinal muscular atrophy type I

190. A child with extremely low birth weight was born 3 months early. An age classification that might help predict potential medical and devopmental problems that might occur after birth is:
    a. Chronologic
    b. Corrected
    c. Gestational
    d. Postconceptional

191. An infant was born at 29 weeks' gestation. This makes the infant extremely vulnerable to light in the neonatal intensive care unit. The reason for this is structural immaturity in the visual system. The structural and functional immaturity that demands that the infant's eyes be shielded from bright lights is:
    a. Eyelids are still fused
    b. Lens are not fully developed
    c. Irises do not constrict significantly
    d. Neurons of the visual cortex are absent

192. A preterm newborn has been diagnosed to have moderate meconium aspiration syndrome (MAS), inadequate oxygenation, and a depressed respiratory drive. Equipment that could be used for oxygen therapy with assisted ventilation would be:

a. Bag and mask ventilation
b. Mechanical ventilation
c. Continuous positive air pressure (CPAP)
d. Extracorporeal membrane oxygenation (ECMO)

193. A visual problem a child with juvenile diabetes is likely to develop is:
    a. Glaucoma
    b. Cataract
    c. Amblyopia
    d. Myopia

194. A 4-year-old has a common pediatric eye disorder, which is blurred vision and external strabismus because the eyeball is too long. The disorder must be corrected with lenses or it can have a significant impact on development. This disorder is:
    a. Hyperopia
    b. Myopia
    c. Astigmatism
    d. Coloboma

195. A 5-year-old was diagnosed with amblyopia 1 year ago. This is a condition of diminished visual acuity. The child has depth perception problems and is often seen tilting their head. Along with treatment, regular assessment is needed to monitor progress of the child's visual acuity. A test that could be administered to assess improvement in visual skills is:
    a. The HOTV test (Matching Test)
    b. The LH Symbols (LEA Symbols)
    c. The Preferential Looking test (PL)
    d. The Snellen vision chart

196. A 5-year-old has severe conductive hearing loss. Diagnoses have determined this was caused by Treacher–Collins syndrome, a hereditary underdevelopment of the external canal and middle ear. Another diagnosis that could lead to conductive hearing loss is:
    a. Otitis media
    b. Hypoxia
    c. Hydrocephalus
    d. Meningitis

197. A 3-year-old child has a hearing impairment. This is caused by meningitis after birth, which resulted in damage to the innermost hair cells of the cochlea. The child misses vowel sounds but hears many consonants. Voices sound weak and thin, but they are understandable if the child is close enough to the speaker. A description of this hearing loss would be:
    a. High-frequency loss

    b. Low-frequency loss
    c. Flat loss
    d. Total loss

198. You have a new 15-year-old patient who presents with rapidly occurring motor and vocal tics that they have been experiencing for more than a year and a half. You suspect:
    a. Tourette's disorder
    b. Substance abuse anxiety disorder
    c. Posttraumatic stress disorder
    d. Conversion disorder

199. An OT has been hired by an agency to address "aging in place with older adults." The therapist would definitely require knowledge and skills related to:
    a. Vocational development
    b. Driving rehabilitation
    c. Environmental adaptation
    d. Leisure pursuits

200. An adolescent was just admitted to your unit with a diagnosis of conduct disorder. The patient is noted to be having problems in home relationships and their grades have taken a turn for the worse. Coming from a MOHO perspective, the MOST appropriate evaluation to use would be:
    a. Kohlman Evaluation of Living Skills (KELS)
    b. Large Allen Cognitive Levels (LACL)
    c. Peabody Developmental Motor Scales (PDMS)
    d. Adolescent Role Assessment

201. You are preparing to evaluate a teenager that was admitted to your unit, using a developmental framework to guide your decision making. The tool would you MOST likely use as part of your evaluation is:
    a. Adolescent Role Assessment
    b. Milwaukee Evaluation of Daily Living Skills (MEDLS)
    c. Learner Magazine Picture Collage
    d. Azima Test Battery

202. When interviewing a mental health client it is important to:
    a. Allow the content of the interview to follow the client's train of thought
    b. Allow your personal feelings to impact the professional relationship that is developing
    c. Remain open and accepting toward the client

d. Stop the interview immediately when any maladaptive behavior occurs

203. During an interview with a new patient on the psychiatric unit, the patient asks if they should divorce their spouse. Your BEST response would be:
    a. "That's not a decision that I can make. I don't know what it is like to be in your situation, but we can talk about it and see if it helps you to make a good decision for yourself."
    b. "Why don't you ask your doctor?"
    c. "Yes. Your spouse seems to be no good from what you have told me. Go ahead and divorce."
    d. "If it were me, I'd dump your spouse."

204. During the evaluation of a patient, the patient says that things are hopeless and "I might as well be dead," as the patient had planned. In this case you would:
    a. Ask some questions to find out more
    b. Tell the patient that those thoughts are stupid
    c. Ignore it and change the subject to something brighter
    d. Tell the patient that you have thought about suicide, too, and that it is normal

205. In a behavioral approach to mental health evaluation and treatment:
    a. The focus is on the past and what made the person misbehave
    b. Maladaptive behaviors are considered the result of faulty learning
    c. Projective techniques are commonly used
    d. The focus is on adapting the environment to support best performance

206. You've decided to use projective techniques in evaluating your patients. It is important to:
    a. Start interpreting their responses in the middle of the session
    b. Get validation from the patient for any information that the process elicits
    c. Use the techniques in a large, open group setting
    d. Run and share your interpretations with the doctor as soon as the patient finishes the task

207. Mentally healthy people:
    a. Should be able to think, feel, and act anyway that they want
    b. Have the psychological make-up to realize their goals
    c. Have never experienced stress in their lives
    d. Know how to manipulate people to get their needs met

208. An 11-year-old is referred for occupational therapy. During observation you note that the client is socially immature and has great difficulty engaging with other kids. You read in the child's chart that for the last 10 years the child lived on a remote island with only their parents for company. The child has never learned to play or interact with children their age. Because of the child's lack of exposure to such normal skill building opportunities, you decide that the BEST framework to use in addressing this case would be:
    a. Cognitive Disabilities Frame of Reference
    b. Cognitive–Behavioral Frame of Reference
    c. Developmental Frame of Reference
    d. Psychoanalytical Frame of Reference

209. A 35-year-old firefighter is admitted to the hospital with severe burns. The patient experiences changes in cognition within a few hours of admission. The patient is confused, disoriented, and having problems focusing their attention. You realize that the patient is probably suffering from:
    a. Amnesia
    b. Delirium
    c. Dementia
    d. Alzheimer's

210. The following statement is true for MOST patients diagnosed with dementia:
    a. The condition is curable and most patients will return to normal functioning
    b. The onset is usually sudden
    c. Substance abuse is a leading cause
    d. The condition is progressive and incurable

211. A patient that you are seeing has come to you with a diagnosis of borderline personality disorder. The axis that you would find noted in this patient's chart is:
    a. Axis I
    b. Axis II
    c. Axis IV
    d. Axis V

212. A disease of the nervous system (not the brain) would be reported under this axis:
    a. Axis I
    b. Axis III
    c. Axis IV
    d. Axis V

213. A patient that has been admitted to your unit has an Axis I diagnosis of dysthymic disorder. You note from previous admissions that the patient also has intellectual disabilities. The axis that the patient's mental retardation is listed under is:
    a. Axis I
    b. Axis II
    c. Axis III
    d. Axis IV

214. A client has experienced recent stresses because of a job loss and its accompanying financial problems. The axis this is reported under is:
    a. Axis II
    b. Axis III
    c. Axis IV
    d. Axis V

215. A patient with a diagnosis of chronic pain is referred to occupational therapy for coping skills related to pain management. Using the cognitive–behavioral approach that addresses thoughts, emotions, and physiology, which technique might the OT used to assist the patient?
    a. Teaching how to follow medication routine
    b. Hypnosis
    c. Thought stopping
    d. Relaxation therapy

216. A client is referred for an occupational therapy evaluation. As you observe the client briefly in the clinic, the patient fluctuates between crying and laughing. You label the patient's affect as:
    a. Labile
    b. Constricted
    c. Bland
    d. Flat

217. A client has been in a fixed position for days and has not responded to others in the environment. The client just sits and stares and does not move. This immobile, constantly maintained position is often seen in:
    a. Catatonia
    b. Mimicry
    c. Mutism
    d. Depression

218. A client comes to your occupational therapy group for the first time and is talking very fast, insists on discussing why their religion is the "one true religion," and reports that they have not slept for

weeks but doesn't need to because they "feel great!" The diagnostic category these symptoms fit in is:
a. Alcohol dependence
b. Major depressive disorder
c. Bipolar disorder I
d. Dysthymic disorder

219. A client has difficulty sticking to the subject in discussions in groups. The client shifts from one idea to another in all conversations. This is known as:
a. Flight of ideas
b. Poverty of thought
c. Blocking
d. Dysthymic disorder

220. Individuals with this diagnosis demonstrate a pervasive pattern of grandiosity, a need for admiration, and a lack of empathy for others. They also may believe that they are exempt from all duties and responsibilities of everyday people. This diagnostic category is:
a. Antisocial personality disorder
b. Avoidant personality disorder
c. Dependent personality disorder
d. Narcissistic personality disorder

221. A college student just relocated to begin a degree program. Two weeks before the patient left home, the patient's significant other of 3 years broke up with them. The patient always thought that they would get married after they graduated. After an intense orientation day for the patient's new school, the patient is found sitting on the floor of their dorm, sobbing uncontrollably, and expressing thoughts of worthlessness and suicidality. Which of the following would be found in the patient's Axis I?
a. Posttraumatic stress disorder
b. Major depression, single episode
c. Life changes; move for college and breakup with significant other
d. Schizophrenia

222. There is an abrupt change in a client's occupational functioning. The client is suddenly unable to walk and reports no feeling from the waist down. Testing identifies no neurologic or orthopedic reason for these symptoms. This is an example of:
a. Tactile hallucinations
b. Conversion symptoms
c. Magical thinking
d. Delusions of grandeur

223. A sixth-grade student seems to panic every time an oral presentation is required in class. The patient reports a fear of being humiliated or embarrassed. This fear disrupts the child's functioning in many school situations. The child is likely struggling with a(n):
    a. Social phobia
    b. Impulse control disorder
    c. Obsessive-compulsive disorder
    d. Antisocial personality disorder

224. A high-powered executive of a Fortune 500 company recently retired because the company offered a substantial early retirement package that the individual could not refuse. After 6 months, the individual gradually began to be less motivated, refusing to get out of bed in the morning, and reported numerous somatic complaints to the family physician, who admitted the individual to the hospital for testing. When referred to the OT for evaluation, the BEST framework to guide the assessment would most likely be:
    a. MOHO
    b. Developmental Frame of Reference
    c. Cognitive Disabilities Frame of Reference
    d. Cognitive–Behavioral Frame of Reference

225. You used the Allen Cognitive Levels (ACL) to evaluate your patient and the person scored a 5.4. A group treatment that would be MOST appropriate for the patient is:
    a. Cooking
    b. Movement
    c. Simple crafts
    d. Grooming

226. You've been asked to evaluate a patient on another unit that the doctor is thinking about discharging. Nursing personnel have expressed some concerns about judgment and decision-making once home. The assessment tool you would choose is:
    a. Work Performance Inventory
    b. Occupational Role History
    c. Kohlman Evaluation Of Living Skills (KELS)
    d. Comprehensive Occupational Therapy Evaluation (COTE)

227. The most life-threatening side effect of antipsychotic medications is:
    a. Tardive dyskinesia
    b. Parkinsonian syndrome
    c. Neuroleptic malignant syndrome
    d. Orthostatic hypotension

228. A 70-year-old patient with mild dementia has moderate difficulty performing instrumental ADLs specifically related to home and money management. An initial assessment should focus on:
    a. Instrumental ADLs
    b. Financial management tasks
    c. Cognitive issues
    d. Home and money management

229. During the intervention review, the OT indicated that the patient has shoulder abduction of a grade of 2. This means that when assessing movement:
    a. Tension can be palpated in the muscles that being tested
    b. The body part moves through partial range in a gravity eliminated position
    c. The body part moves through the full range in a gravity eliminated position
    d. The body part moves less than full range against gravity

230. An OT is administering a sensory test to a patient with an ulnar nerve injury. The initial step in performing the test begins by:
    a. Applying the stimulus to the affected area with vision occluded
    b. Applying the stimulus to the affected area without occluding vision
    c. Establishing an area that tests within normal limits
    d. Mapping the distribution of the peripheral nerves in the extremity

231. The OT is asked to perform a home assessment for an individual prior to discharge from skilled nursing care. The initial step in the process is:
    a. Interview family members and friends who may take part in the individual's care
    b. Identify the roles and occupational tasks the individual will be performing
    c. Identify obstacles that would interfere with easy mobilization and access to the home
    d. Access mobility issues that may interfere with the individual's occupational performance

232. A 6-year-old elementary school child has a problem with handwriting. The child demonstrates gaps in handwriting skills that could improve with a comprehensive, repetitive program that focuses on the acquisition of these skills. A behavior the child should exhibit at this stage to improve handwriting is:

    a. At the acquisition stage, a child observes the behavior of others and determines the consequences, and these observations are stored in memory for later use

    b. The child may decide to perform the behavior, depending on the child's perception of the situation and the consequences

    d. The child learns through experiences (e.g., problem solving) in situations in which a child, an activity, and an adult are components

    d. The child may take the initiative to observe other children performing the same task and practice until skill is mastered

233. In an inpatient setting, assessments of individuals with a diagnosis of traumatic brain injury often begin with:
    a. Instrumental ADLs
    b. Basic ADL skills
    c. Visual screens, perception, and cognition
    d. Mobility

234. A patient with deep partial thickness burns has an extremely edematous right arm with some open wound areas still visible. The OT wants to assess the effectiveness of the treatment in reducing the amount of swelling present. The BEST approach is to:
    a. Use a volumeter
    b. Assess pain level before and after treatment
    c. Do circumferential measurements
    d. Ask the patient if the extremity feels lighter

235. The OT receives a referral to treat a 45-year-old patient diagnosed with lung cancer that has metastasized to the brain. The physician asked that the patient be seen that day because the patient is scheduled to receive radiation treatment in the afternoon. When the therapist approaches the patient, they refuse to be seen because insurance coverage has run out and the patient cannot afford to pay for treatment. Responding consistently with the Code of Ethics, the OT will MOST likely:
    a. Treat the patient per the physician order and notify the nurse of the situation
    b. Not treat the patient based on the refusal and document interaction in the chart
    c. Treat the patient but do not charge or document the service provision

    d.   Not treat the patient but charge for the time spent reviewing medical records

236. An important FIRST step to perform for a patient who is in need of a program for dysphagia is to examine:
    a.   Ability to bring food to the mouth for self-feeding
    b.   Oral and pharyngeal control, motion, and sensation
    c.   Which texture of food will work best for eating
    d.   The type of adaptive utensil to use

237. A provocative test that is sometime used to determined the presence of carpal tunnel syndrome is the:
    a.   Finklestein test
    b.   Froment sign
    c.   Ligamentous instability test
    d.   Phalen sign

238. When administering a standardized test, the BEST strategy for the therapist to follow is to:
    a.   Modify the testing instructions as needed
    b.   Use two persons to administer the test for consistency
    c.   Follow the testing procedures as stated
    d.   Administer testing procedures over two sessions

239. Before providing intervention, the OT must establish baseline data on the individual's level of endurance. An objective method to measure endurance is:
    a.   Asking the patient to rate the level of fatigue on a scale of 1–10
    b.   The number of repetition of an activity per unit of time
    c.   Using clinical observation to note change in rate of response
    d.   Taking blood pressure before and after an activity

240. Two therapists administered a test approximately 1 week apart that assessed fine motor prehension skills in a patient. The test results showed no change in the individual status between the first and last testing session. This would indicate that the test instrument has:
    a.   Internal validity
    b.   External validity
    c.   High reliability
    d.   Low reliability

241. An instrument/technique the OT might choose to assess moving two-point discrimination of a client with sensory deficits in the fingers is:
    a.   Monofilament test
    b.   A paper clip
    c.   Disk criminator
    d.   Stereognosis test

242. The OT wishes to assess if the patient can detect and identify placement of parts of the body and body positions with the vision occluded. The sensorimotor component being evaluated is:
    a. Kinesthesia
    b. Proprioception
    c. Functional mobility
    d. Postural control

243. In testing for a patient's ability to identify numbers or letters by tracing shapes on the surface of the skin, the therapist is assessing:
    a. Stereognosis
    b. Graphesthesia
    c. Form constancy
    d. Visual closure

244. The OT is evaluating a child with mild spastic diplegia. A performance deficit that is important to assess is:
    a. Tactile defensiveness
    b. Gravitational insecurity
    c. Postural insecurity
    d. Overresponsiveness

245. A 10-year-old child in the third grade has age-appropriate reading and writing abilities but deficits when performing simple subtraction and addition problems. The child also has difficulty solving problems that involve multiple steps or columns. To assist this child with these performance deficits, the OT should assess:
    a. Visual memory and spatial relations
    b. Visual-discrimination problems
    c. Object (form) problems
    d. Visual acuity

246. A functional reach screen conducted by the OT shows that the client is unable to move body parts independent of each other. The NEXT area to assess is:
    a. Endurance
    b. Standing balance
    c. Strength
    d. Postural control

247. The OT completes an occupational profile on a 16-year-old with juvenile rheumatoid arthritis. Using scientific reasoning, the NEXT step in the process is:
    a. Identify goals and concerns of the client
    b. Administer a functional motion assessment

   c. Develop treatment goals and timelines

   d. Identify activities for intervention

248. The OT administered a visual perceptual assessment tool to a patient with Bell's palsy degeneration at the beginning of therapy and prior to the family-rehab team meeting. Administering an assessment tool in this fashion measures:
   a. Inter-rater reliability
   b. Test-retest reliability
   c. Standard error of measurement
   d. Central tendency

249. The OT wants to observe the dynamic balance of a client. An activity the therapist could use to observe this skill is:
   a. Transferring in and out of the bathtub/shower
   b. Putting on a shirt over head
   c. Throwing a ball
   d. Driving a car

250. An activity that would be contraindicated for an arthritic patient using principles of joint protection with lifting is:
   a. Pushing or sliding items along kitchen counter
   b. Changing position often when working
   c. Storing frequently used items with in easy reach
   d. Carrying items in hands whenever possible

251. An OT administers a standardized test to assess fine motor coordination patterns and speed of manipulation in a patient with rheumatoid arthritis. One method to determine if the patient's performance on the test is within normal limits is to:
   a. Compare the scores with the normative data available
   b. Perform test-retest procedures on the patient
   c. Record clinical observations on patient's performance while testing
   d. Compare scores to a similar standardized assessment

252. What processing deficit might the OT need to address in a patient with advanced chronic obstructive pulmonary disease?
   a. Confusion
   b. Recognition
   c. Memory loss
   d. Categorization

253. A patient presents in the outpatient rehabilitation clinic with deficits in trunk and upper extremity weakness affecting dynamic sitting balance. In this case, the BEST testing procedure to use to evaluate occupational performance skills and deficits would be:
   a. Clinical observation

   b. Standardized testing

   c. Non-standardized testing

   d. Functional motion assessment

254. A typical psychosocial response that may be seen in a patient with HIV/AIDS that will also have influence on treatment is:
   a. Mourning
   b. Manic episodes
   c. Increased socializations
   d. Manic-depressive episodes

255. A patient with a diagnosis of agnosia should be assessed in the area of:
   a. Motor apraxia
   b. Visual and tactile perception
   c. Swallowing
   d. Postural control

256. A patient with lymphedema is prescribed a resting hand splint to maintain joint alignment and functional positioning. The BEST method the OT could use is:
   a. A splint secured with a bandage wrapped circumferentially
   b. A splint with narrow straps secured at the position of the forearm, wrist, and hand
   c. A splint with wide straps secured at the position of the forearm, wrist, and hand
   d. A circumferential cast

257. A client presents with depressive symptoms, a possible personality disorder, and chronic back pain. The axis that you would find the chronic back pain listed under is:
   a. Axis I
   b. Axis II
   c. Axis III
   d. Axis IV

258. During an interview, the OT discovers that a 77-year-old client is having difficulty recalling tasks that they need to perform while engaging in their volunteer work. Based on this information, the assessment should include the:
   a. Kohlman Evaluation of Living Skills
   b. ACL
   c. Role checklist
   d. Interest checklist

259. A new patient has just been brought to the psychiatric unit and you cannot understand anything the patient is saying. Every fifth word

that the patient speaks seems to be in English. Your NEXT step would be:

a. Find an interpreter that can translate
b. Go back to the patient's chart and see if there are any notations addressing this behavior
c. Give the patient a craft project to do and see how the patient performs
d. Discharge the patient from your caseload, because you cannot help

260. A 21-year-old patient was admitted following a suicide attempt. In your first conversation the patient expresses some worry over missing their college classes while in the hospital. The BEST next step for you is to:

a. Contact the patient's teachers to let them know that the patient is in a psychiatric hospital
b. Encourage the student to contact the teachers and inform them about class attendance
c. Call the patient's parents and have them call the patient's teachers to tell them that the patient is in the psychiatric hospital, so that you do not break confidentiality
d. Tell the patient to withdraw from the patient's classes to get rid of the stress

261. The OT has been working to improve the memory of a client on the mental health unit who exhibits mild cognitive deficits. Initially, the client was asked to identify the names of several common household objects, which they have mastered. To progress this patient, the NEXT step for the OT is to:

a. Introduce several more new items
b. Work on regrouping of the same items
c. Require that the patient spell all items
d. Ask the patient to locate the old items among several new items

262. An elderly client has been brought to your unit for evaluation. The client has obvious cognitive deficits that impair social and occupational functioning. The client's child tells the team that these problems have been developing gradually over a long period of time, and that the client just continues to get worse. You suspect:

a. A head injury
b. Alzheimer's
c. Major depression
d. Substance-induced amnestic disorder

263. In psychiatric practice it is considered a "dual diagnosis" when the patient:

a. Presents with two separate psychotic disorders.
b. Presents with a heart condition and a mental problem.

    c. Presents with a substance abuse problem and a psychiatric diagnosis.

    d. Has been admitted two different times and under two different diagnoses.

264. A person with a long history of substance abuse who develops Korsakoff's syndrome is likely to:

    a. Confabulate to fill in memory gaps

    b. Start using heroin

    c. Develop tardive dyskinesia

    d. Develop tics

265. Trichotillomania is a condition that involves:

    a. Pulling out one's own hair

    b. Getting hysterical when someone tickles you

    c. Getting hysterical when someone frightens you

    d. Fainting at the sight of blood

266. A low score on the COTE means that the patient:

    a. Is low functioning and needs a great deal of OT intervention

    b. Has a poor memory

    c. Is high functioning and needs limited OT intervention

    d. Has severe motor difficulties

267. An OT using relaxation training would MOST likely be addressing person with:

    a. Manic-depressive disorder

    b. Depression

    c. Schizophrenia

    d. Anxiety

268. You are trying to interview a client, but the client constantly changes the subject and it seems that a single word can trigger the client's conversation to take an entirely new direction. This behavior is known as:

    a. Confusion

    b. Flight of ideas

    c. Psychosis

    d. Delusions

269. A disorder that involves a client intentionally causing their body harm to produce physical symptoms of illness or injury to fulfill their psychological need for attention from medical personnel is:

    a. Narcolepsy

    b. Pedophilia

    c. Munchausen's

    d. Voyeurism

270. A treatment used with patients as a last resort and involves using electricity causing a patient to have a seizure is:
    a. Electroconvulsive therapy
    b. Insulin therapy
    c. Cryogenics
    d. Hypnosis

271. A patient on an inpatient psychiatric unit has to be watched closely because they tend to drink water excessively. In fact, the patient has been known to turn the water on in the shower and place their mouth under the faucet to drink. This type of behavior is associated with a condition called:
    a. Polycytosis
    b. Polydipsia
    c. Polymyalgia
    d. Hyperemesis

272. You have been asked to see a profoundly mentally handicapped individual for occupational therapy services. You can expect that the client will be:
    a. Able to feed and dress independently
    b. Dependent on others for personal care
    c. Able to carry on simple conversations using complex sentences
    d. Able to complete household chore with minimal assist

273. A situation in which an OT would not directly address the psychological needs of a client is when they are treating a:
    a. Patient with learning disabilities
    c. Patient with rheumatoid arthritis
    c. Patient with autism
    d. Comatose patient

274. A school-based evaluation of a first-grader's handwriting should always include:
    a. Administering the Development Test of Visual-Motor Integration
    b. Administering the Motor Free Visual Perceptual Test
    c. Observing the child write on an inclined surface
    d. Observing the child write in a natural setting

275. Sensory defensiveness, gravitational insecurity, aversive response to movement, and poor registration are associated with:
    a. Poor sensory modulation
    b. Poor kinesthesia
    c. Dyspraxia
    d. Poor bilateral integration and sequencing

276. During an assessment of developmental play, the OT determines that a child has accurate and direct reaching abilities and can grasp with the fingertips. The child also plays with toys at the midline, can bang objects together, and release them into a container. The NEXT skill for the OT to assess is to determine if the child can:
    a. Assemble a 4- to 5-piece puzzle
    b. Use one hand while the other manipulates
    c. Draw with crayons
    d. Snip with scissors and turn pages

277. If a school-based OT is interested in evaluating the amount of assistance a middle school student requires and their performance for tasks, such as eating and drinking, clothing management, and written work, the MOST appropriate assessment would be:
    a. Adolescent/Adult Sensory Profile
    b. School Function Assessment
    c. Bruininks–Oseretsky Test of Motor Proficiency
    d. Functional Independence Measure for Children

278. A student described as underresponsive or presenting with a high neurologic threshold on the Sensory Profile may display the following behavior at school:
    a. Risk-taking behavior, such as jumping off playground equipment
    b. Difficulty copying from the board
    c. Fear of playground equipment or sports
    d. Moving or pulling away from unexpected touch

279. A school-based OT evaluating a student with autism may anticipate observing all of the following behaviors, except:
    a. Limited social interaction, such as limited eye contact
    b. Limited communication, such as echolalic speech
    c. Altered growth, including specific facial features
    d. Unconventional behaviors, such as rocking, spinning, or hand-flapping

280. Non-standardized observations used to assess sensory integration in a school-based setting may include the following, except:
    a. Stereognosis and touch localization
    b. Prone extension and supine flexion
    c. Crossing midline and hand preference
    d. Sequential finger touching and finger to nose

281. You are evaluating a 55-year-old patient with ALS who is nonambulatory (now using a power wheelchair) and has significant arm weakness. At this time the patient's deficit areas are limited to

lower motor neuron deficits. An area of occupation that should be addressed is:

a. Dressing
b. Feeding
c. Health management and maintenance
d. Care of pets

Answers to Evaluation Questions

1. a. A family is referred for an early intervention screening at which a developmental therapist or OT screens the child to determine if a full assessment is necessary. *Pediatric Occupational Therapy and Early Intervention* by Case-Smith

2. a. Daily living skills in infants refer to self-sustaining skills, such as feeding and sleeping. Sleep patterns can be evaluated from the parent's description of a typical day. Daily living skills also refer to bathing and dressing, but this is as it involves the parents. *Pediatric Occupational Therapy and Early Intervention* by Case-Smith

3. d. Although therapists suggest goals based on the evaluation process, ultimately a child's parents decide which goals will be included and which goals are a priority. Goals that relate specifically to the family's concerns about the care of their child are included in the plan. If therapists have other goals, these can be added with parental consent. *Pediatric Occupational Therapy and Early Intervention* by Case-Smith

4. c. Children with known chromosomal, structural, or metabolic defects are classified as having established risk. *Pediatric Occupational Therapy and Early Intervention* by Case-Smith

5. a. A child experiencing sensory defensiveness has a tendency to respond negatively to sensation that is considered by most people to be noninvasive or nonirritating. This frequently includes hyperresponsiveness to light or unexpected touches, high-frequency noises, certain visual stimulation, or certain smells and tastes. *Sensory Integration: Theory and Practice* by Bundy

6. c. The Peabody assesses a child's abilities with gross and fine motor skills. *Occupational Therapy for Children* by Case-Smith

7. b. Persons with long-standing diabetes frequently have increased incidences of other conditions, such as peripheral neuropathies. Therefore, a sensory evaluation is necessary to determine if sensation is diminished. A person with diminished sensation secondary to peripheral neuropathy may not be able to perceive or gauge pressure when wearing a splint. This can lead to skin breakdown. *Introduction to Splinting: A Clinical Reasoning & Problem Solving Process* by Coppard and Lohman

8. b. A norm-referenced test is developed by giving the test in question to a large number of children, usually several hundred or more. This group is the normative group and norms or averages are derived from this sample. When a norm-referenced test is administered, the performance of the child being tested is compared to the normative sample. *Occupational Therapy for Children* by Case-Smith

9. d. The day, month, and year of the child's birth date is subtracted from the date of testing. *Occupational Therapy for Children* by Case-Smith

10. a. Corrected age is used for children who were born prematurely to "correct" for the number of weeks they were born before the due date. Generally the age is corrected until the child turns 2 years old. Many practitioners consider 36 to 37 weeks and above to be full-term gestation. Children with a gestation period of 36 weeks and above do not receive a corrected age. Subtract the birth date from the due date to yield the exact measurement of prematurity, and to calculate the corrected age, subtract the amount of prematurity from the chronologic age. *Occupational Therapy for Children* by Case-Smith

11. a. The team dealing with the case should use lay terminology to describe the early intervention process and repeat information to make sure that the parents understand. They should also welcome parental feedback and incorporate the parents' ideas into a suggested activity. Professionals should encourage parents to ask questions and repeat information when necessary. Because the language used by health care professionals is often technical and medically related, families can easily misunderstand its meaning. OTs and other team members must make a concerted effort to use lay terminology to describe function, rather than neurophysiologic components. *Occupational Therapy for Children* by Case-Smith

12. b. This stage is characterized by holding on and letting go and is exemplified by the crisis that occurs through the toilet-training process. This stage brings independent movement away from the parents, enabling the child to explore the environment. Parents must provide opportunities for the child to make choices and develop a sense of self-controlled will. *Occupational Therapy for Children* by Case-Smith

13. a. Assimilation is the reception of sensory stimuli from internal and external environments. Accommodation is the motor

response to these stimuli. Association is the organized process of relating current sensory information with the current motor response and then relating this relationship to past responses. Differentiation is the process of identifying the specific elements in a situation that are useful and relevant to another situation to refine the responsive pattern. *Occupational Therapy for Children* by Case-Smith

14.   b.   A child diagnosed with mental retardation will show significantly impaired intellectual ability, behavioral deficits, and impairment of the skills required for independence in occupational performance areas (i.e., age-appropriate play, dressing, and communication). *Occupational Therapy for Children* by Case-Smith

15.   b.   In lead poisoning, lead affects the circulatory system by severely limiting the body's ability to synthesize heme, leading to the accumulation of alternate metabolites in the body and, ultimately, anemia. The most significant and irreversible damage occurs in the nervous system. Fluid builds up in the brain, and intracranial pressure can reach life-threatening levels. Cortical atrophy and lead encephalitis can lead to mental retardation, paralysis, blindness, and deafness. *Occupational Therapy for Children* by Case-Smith

16.   d.   In diplegia, the lower extremities are impaired significantly, with only mild involvement of the upper extremities. Hemiplegia involves the impairment of upper and lower limbs on one side of the body, and tetraplegia or quadriplegia means that all four extremities are affected. Therefore, diplegia is the possible classification of the child's condition. *Occupational Therapy for Children* by Case-Smith

17.   d.   Although researchers are still struggling to find conclusive evidence for the etiology of ADHD, studies have demonstrated that ADHD runs in families and three genes have been found to be related to ADHD implicating genetic factors. Imaging in individuals with ADHD has shown decreased activity in the frontal parietal lobes, which inhibit impulsiveness, pointing to neurologic factors. Medications that influence neurotransmitter function are effective in treatment of ADHD, indicating neurochemical imbalances. *Occupational Therapy for Children* by Case-Smith

18.   b.   Tourette's syndrome is a pervasive disorder that affects neurologic and motor behavioral function, especially motor tics and vocalizations. Therefore, it is likely that the child has

Tourette's syndrome. *Occupational Therapy for Children* by Case-Smith

19. c. Chemotherapy is administered in phase III—the intensification and consolidation phase—to remove small deposits of cells that remain after remission. *Occupational Therapy for Children* by Case-Smith

20. a. Duchenne's muscular dystrophy is an X-linked recessive disorder caused by the deficiency in the production of dystrophin. Dystrophin is a component of the plasma membrane of the muscle fibers, the deficiency of which causes the muscle to degenerate and malfunction. The calf muscles are enlarged because of fibrosis and proliferation of the adipose tissue, which causes muscle weakness. Therefore, the child's condition could be diagnosed as Duchenne's muscular dystrophy. *Occupational Therapy for Children* by Case-Smith

21. a. Disturbances in communication can range from mild (slight articulation impairment) to severe (muteness); thus, the more mild the communication deficit, the more likely the child will develop sufficient communication to function as an adult. *Occupational Therapy for Children* by Case-Smith

22. a. Oral motor deficits relate to issues with the oral motor musculature around the mouth. OTs are qualified to address deficits related to swallowing or dysphagia, chewing, and drooling. *Occupational Therapy for Children* by Case-Smith

23. c. The teacher has already identified the child as being at risk for developmental or functional deficits. Therefore, it is appropriate to use a type II assessment, which is the Short Sensory Profile. This caregiver questionnaire measures the frequency of behaviors related to sensory processing, modulation, and emotional responsivity to sensory input in children 3 to 12 years of age. The Ages & Stages Questionnaires, First STEp, and the Denver-II pertain to the early screening to identify children at risk for disabilities. *Occupational Therapy for Children* by Case-Smith

24. d. The School Function Assessment is a judgment-based questionnaire designed to measure a student's performance of functional tasks that support his or her participation in the academic and social aspects of an elementary school program (kindergarten through grade 6). Three scales evaluate the student's level of participation, the type and amount of task supports needed, and his or her activity performance on

specific school tasks. *Occupational Therapy for Children* by Case-Smith

25. c. According to the Standards of Practice for Occupational Therapy, an OTA would perform functions such as administering some of the assessments and documenting some of the results. Selecting evaluation methods and measures, interpreting and analyzing assessment data, and writing goals are functions of the OT. *Occupational Therapy for Children* by Case-Smith

26. b. The child needs to undergo PDMS-2. PDMS-2 tests the domains such as gross motor scale and fine motor scale and uses the standard scores such as T scores, Z scores, and Developmental Motor Quotient scores. *Occupational Therapy for Children* by Case-Smith

27. d. In flexion reactions, the infant can maintain head alignment with the body without the initial head lag when pulled to a sitting position. In the neck on body reaction, the infant can turn the head to the sides giving a segmental roll response. The Landau reactions are observed in prone suspension position and not supine and sitting position. The body on head reaction is observed in the prone position on a support level. *Occupational Therapy for Children* by Case-Smith

28. c. Children with limited anticipatory postural control have difficulty catching, reaching, or throwing in any posture, as a result of a poor feed-forward control. Protective reactions are mainly to protect the infant from a fall. A problem with development of higher-level balance skills is evidenced by inability to stand on one limb, walk on balance beam, or hop. *Occupational Therapy for Children* by Case-Smith

29. c. In eyes closed, swayed-reference platform, and swayed-referenced visual surround and platform, the child needs to rely only on vestibular information, without any visual or somatosensory cues. In eyes closed, stable platform and eyes open, swayed-reference platform, there is visual input with inaccurate somatosensory cues, and the child does not completely rely on vestibular function. *Occupational Therapy for Children* by Case-Smith

30. a. According to the PDMS, most children can cut across a 6-inch piece of paper by the age of 2½ years. By 3 to 3½ years of age, they can cut on a line that is 6 inches long. By 3½ to 4 years of

age, they can cut a circle. By 4½ to 5 years of age, they can cut a square. *Occupational Therapy for Children* by Case-Smith

31. c. This issue needs attention first. The child's inability to maintain the sitting position without supporting with one arm limits the patient's ability to engage in bilateral activities and may interfere with the development of grasp, release, and object manipulation skills. Limitations in trunk movement and control may be caused by a central nervous system dysfunction or generalized muscle weakness. *Occupational Therapy for Children* by Case-Smith

32. c. By 8–9 months of age, visual-motor coordination is more refined, and the infant differentiates thumb and finger movements to hold objects with an opposed grasp. *Occupational Therapy for Children* by Case-Smith

33. b. The power grasp often is used to control tools or other objects. The hook grasp is used when strength of grasp must be maintained to carry objects. Lateral pinch is used to exert power on or with a small object. Opposition of the thumb tip and the tip of the index finger, forming a circle, describes the tip pinch which is used to get small objects. *Occupational Therapy for Children* by Case-Smith

34. c. The OT can observe the child's ability to sequence shoulder, elbow, wrist, and finger movements, while stabilizing the arm against gravity. *Occupational Therapy for Children* by Case-Smith

35. b. The biomechanical frame of reference is used in assessing and treating children with limitations in ROM, strength, or endurance that affect their hand skills. It is used to explain difficulties in arm use for reach caused by problems in postural alignment or impaired ability to use the arms against gravity. *Occupational Therapy for Children* by Case-Smith

36. a. Limited finger isolation and control and the inability to hold more than one object in the hand at the same time are two of the problems that limit in-hand manipulation. Praxis and motor control problems, particularly of the intrinsic muscles, may be a major cause of such limited in-hand manipulation skill development. Difficulty with sustained arm position during object placement and release and difficulty combining wrist extension with finger extension are not problems that limit in-hand manipulation but affect voluntary release skills that

depend on control of arm and finger movement. *Occupational Therapy for Children* by Case-Smith

37. d. One of the commonly observed sensory integrative dysfunctions involving sensory modulation is tactile defensiveness. It is a tendency to overreact to ordinary touch sensations that most people do not find bothersome. Common irritants include certain textures of clothing, grass or sand against bare skin, and glue or paint. The child is therefore tactually defensive. Being aware of the specific textures and tactile inputs that she is averse to would help you identify a strategy to help her cope with her problem. *Occupational Therapy for Children* by Case-Smith

38. d. Children with problems in discriminating vestibular proprioceptive stimuli may face difficulties in knowing the position of the body in space and its relationship to surroundings. They are unable to judge the right force to be used for activities such as writing or clapping. Difficulty in perceiving form and space and relationship among objects, and difficulty perceiving depth, distance, location of boundaries, and space between objects is observed in children having problems discriminating visual stimuli. *Occupational Therapy for Children* by Case-Smith

39. a. Children with sensory integrative disorder are oversensitive to touch, movement, sights, and sounds. They may also have delays in speech, language, and other motor skills. Being inattentive, impulsive, and hyperactive are signs that point toward ADHD rather than sensory integrative disorder. *Occupational Therapy for Children* by Case-Smith

40. c. At 1–2 years of age, discrimination and localization of tactile sensations become much more precise, allowing for further refinement of fine motor skills. This is because throughout the second year, the typically developing toddler experiments with many variations in body movements. During the second 6 months, the child learns about environmental space and about the body's relationship to external space through sensorimotor experiences. At 3–7 years of age, sensorimotor functions become consolidated as a foundation for higher intellectual abilities. This is a crucial period for sensory integration. During the first 6 months of the first year, the infant begins to show a strong inner drive to rise up against gravity. *Occupational Therapy for Children* by Case-Smith

41. c. Children with mild spastic diplegia usually have postural insecurity. These children typically react with anxiety when faced with a minimal climbing task. They may show pleasure when the head is radically tilted in different planes as long as they are securely held. Tactile defensiveness is a tendency to overreact to ordinary touch sensations. Children who display gravitational insecurity often show signs of inordinate fear, anxiety, or avoidance in relation to stairs, escalators, or elevators; moving or high pieces of playground equipment; and uneven or unpredictable surfaces. A child who is overresponsive is overwhelmed by ordinary sensory input and reacts defensively to it, often with strong negative emotions and activation of the sympathetic nervous system. *Occupational Therapy for Children* by Case-Smith

42. b. A tendency to generate responses that are appropriately graded in relation to incoming sensory stimuli, rather than underreacting or overreacting to them, is called sensory modulation. Sensory registration is the ability to register and attend to relevant environmental stimuli. Some children register sensations yet are underresponsive to the incoming stimuli and seem to seek intense stimulation in the sensory modalities that are affected. Such behavior is called sensation seeking behavior. Sensory discrimination allows for refined organization and interpretation of sensory stimuli. *Occupational Therapy for Children* by Case-Smith

43. a. In strabismus, an eye overtly turns in, out, up, or down because of muscular imbalance causing double vision or mental suppression of one of the images. In a phoric condition, overt misalignment of the two eyes is absent and myopia is shortsightedness. In astigmatism, the patient experiences blurred vision at distances both near and far. *Occupational Therapy for Children* by Case-Smith

44. d. Children with visual–spatial problems have difficulty in correctly aligning the columns for math problems. Therefore, the answers are incorrect because of alignment and not because of calculation skills. In visual–spatial problems, the child has problems with handwriting. The child may reverse the letters and numbers. In visual–discrimination problems, the child has difficulty identifying letters and numbers. Object (form) problems include form constancy, visual closure, and figure-ground. This affects the visual identification of objects by color, texture, shape, and size. *Occupational Therapy for Children* by Case-Smith

45.   a.   Depth perception is an ability to determine the relative distance between objects. This perceptual ability provides an awareness of how far away something is. This assists the hand to orient properly for grasping. Problems with depth perception may affect the orientation of the hand for grasping before reaching. *Occupational Therapy for Children* by Case-Smith

46.   b.   The child could have a spatial vision problem and an impairment of ocular mobility. A child with spatial vision problems is not able copy properly from the blackboard and is typically a poor speller. The child also complains of his eyes being tired, so he may have an impairment of ocular mobility. A child with diminished topographic orientation is unable to find his or her way from one location to another. In visual discrimination problems, the child is not able to recognize words or symbols and therefore is slow in mastering the alphabet or numbers. *Occupational Therapy for Children* by Case-Smith

47.   c.   Selective attention is the ability to choose relevant visual information while ignoring less relevant information. It is conscious, focused attention. This child is unable to do that. Therefore, the child may have difficulty with selective attention. Children with visual memory problems are unable to remember the shape of letters and words. A child with divided attention difficulty is not able to respond to two or more task. Alertness is a transition from a state of being awake to being attentive. *Occupational Therapy for Children* by Case-Smith

48.   d.   Research shows that about 40% of school-aged children remember visually-presented information, whereas only 20% to 30% recall what is heard. A child in the age group of 6–7 years would prefer kinesthetic input to learn effectively. They learn easily through the whole-body movements. Tactile input channels develop a child's first perceptions of the world. *Occupational Therapy for Children* by Case-Smith

49.   b.   A slow to warm up child is shy and passive and transitions are often problematic for such a child. A slow to warm up child shows negative reactions to new stimuli and is slow in adapting to new and changing situations. An easy child is positive in mood and adapts effectively to new situations and demands. The difficult child is unpredictable, withdrawing, non-adaptive to changes, and extremely negative and intense. *Occupational Therapy for Children* by Case-Smith

50. a. The symptoms and signs exhibited by this child are characteristics of major depression, which is a subcategory of mood disorder. Anxiety disorder is characterized by fearfulness and feelings of unease. Bipolar disorder is characterized by manic behavior. Mood disorders involve long-term changes in the child's prevailing emotions. *Occupational Therapy for Children* by Case-Smith

51. b. Forgetfulness, impulsiveness, and leaving the task unfinished are characteristics observed with ADHD. Therefore, this child may have ADHD. In obsessive-compulsive disorder, the child does an activity again and again or attends overly much to detail and precision. In PDD, restricted, repetitive, and stereotyped patterns of behavior, interests, and activities are often observed. However, delayed or missing speech, language, and nonverbal communication skills are also present. *Occupational Therapy for Children* by Case-Smith

52. d. Principles for testing sensation include occluding the vision and applying the stimulus in an irregular pattern to the involved area, or areas representing the distribution of the nerve. *Occupational Therapy for Physical Dysfunction* by Trombly and Radomski

53. d. The goals of early therapy are to normalize edema and achieve AROM of area that are not casted. One complication of casting is intrinsic and extrinsic muscle tightness. Tendon gliding exercises and passive ROM are two gentle techniques that are useful in providing early mobilization with fractures. *Occupational Therapy for Physical Dysfunction* by Trombly and Radomski

54. a. Narrative reasoning is a client-centered approach that encourages the individual to share their story, history, concerns, and goals. This approach can assist in understanding habits, routines, roles, and how the illness or condition has affected one's occupational performance, which are all parts of the occupational profile. *Occupational Therapy for Physical Dysfunction* by Trombly and Radomski

55. d. An intervention review is a formal continuous process that assesses a client's progress. Intervention review identifies the effectiveness of the interventions and the progress toward targeted outcomes. *Applying the Occupational Therapy Practice Framework* by Skubik-Peplaski, Paris, Boyle, and Culpert

56. a. Evaluation of a client's AROM provides the OT with preliminary information regarding muscle strength. With a fair minus grade, the body part moves less than full range through the arc of motion against gravity. The client must have a fair grade to achieve AROM against gravity. Resistance is applied to assess a "good" grade, and poor muscle grade requires gravity to be eliminated and no resistance to achieve the full range. *Occupational Therapy for Physical Dysfunction* by Trombly and Radomski

57. d. The occupational profile is a means of gathering preliminary data on the client's history, roles, routines, habits, and goals. The information obtained guides the evaluation process. Using a client-centered approach, a written inventory designed to capture the information needed would be the most appropriate strategy. Deafness does not hinder using other forms of communication. Although a family member can provide some information, the goal is to involve the patient as much as possible in the process. A standardized test and home visit to observe the person in action are essentially assessments that according to the *OT Practice Framework* come after the development of the occupational profile. *Applying the Occupational Therapy Practice Framework* by Skubik-Peplaski, Paris, Boyle, and Culpert

58. d. Dyspraxia (praxis) refers to the inability to follow through with nonhabitual motor acts. Children who exhibit this condition will have difficulty attaining basic skills that other children can easily perform, such as jumping rope, completing a puzzle, or in more severe cases, self-feeding and dressing. *Occupational Therapy for Children* by Case-Smith

59. a. The radial nerve produces the symptoms involved in this scenario and the distribution of that nerve is the posterior elbow, forearm, and dorsal-lateral aspect of the hand; therefore, sensory and motor issues will occur in these areas. The OT should assess and plot sensory return based on the nerve distribution. *Occupational Therapy for Physical Dysfunction* by Trombly and Radomski

60. c. Spinal cord injuries usually do not have associated change in cognitive function. A patient with a spinal cord injury at the level of C6 would exhibit either significant difficulties or total lack of function with all of the areas listed except cognition. *Basic Rehabilitation Techniques: A Self Instructional Guide* by Sine, Liss, Roush, Holcomb, and Wilson

61. a. Functional outcomes of a C7 spinal cord lesion are independence in mobility with a manual or powered wheelchair, independence in transfers with adapted devices or a sliding board, and independence in ADLs with adapted equipment. *Basic Rehabilitation Techniques: A Self Instructional Guide* by Sine, Liss, Roush, Holcomb, and Wilson

62. b. A person who lacks sensation tends to grips with excessive pressure, which can lead to bruising and decubiti. Decubiti and bruising in someone with diabetes may lead to serious issues related to tissue healing. *Basic Rehabilitation Techniques: A Self Instructional Guide* by Sine, Liss, Roush, Holcomb, and Wilson

63. c. Dysphasia or swallowing problems are common with head and neck cancer. With chemotherapy, edema may occur and reduce salivary flow. Other issues may involve decreased tongue movements that would also affect swallowing. *Occupational Therapy for Physical Dysfunction* by Trombly and Radomski

64. b. As a first step, the team must develop a comprehensive description of the problem, including individual and environmental factors that influence the issue, and they should define the problem clearly and objectively. The team members should then make a commitment to solving the problem. *Occupational Therapy for Children* by Case-Smith

65. a. Norm-referenced tests are developed by giving the test to a large sample of persons with similar characteristics or in a similar setting. The group is called the normative sample, the norms or average scores that are derived from the population. Norm-referenced tests compare the person being tested to the average performance of the normative sample. *Occupational Therapy Practice Skills for Physical Dysfunction* by Pedretti and Early

66. c. Resistance such as manual muscle testing can compromise or further injure a site that has recently undergone surgery. Any resistive activity or assessment will require physician's approval before initiating. *Occupational Therapy Practice Skills for Physical Dysfunction* by Pedretti and Early

67. d. In the case of a shoulder impingement, movement overhead, as in putting on an overhead garment, may cause the joint space to narrow, causing increased pressure and possible discomfort to the structures of the shoulder joint. *Occupational Therapy: Practice Skills for Physical Dysfunction* by Pedretti and Early

68. a. Tapping over the nerve 4–6 weeks after an injury can elicit shocking and shooting sensations distal to the site of suture and

signal regrowth of a nerve. *Hand & Upper Extremity Rehabilitation* by Burke, Higgins, McClinton, Saunders, and Valdata

69. b. Monofilament tests are used to measure touch pressure threshold that detects the degree of sensory return. Monofilaments are also a good tool to use for sensory mapping and plotting sensory return. The filaments range in different sizes and can detect sensory return ranging from normal, impaired light touch, impaired protective sensation, and loss of sensation to being undetectable. *Hand & Upper Extremity Rehabilitation* by Burke, Higgins, McClinton, Saunders, and Valdata

70. c. In cardiac rehabilitation protocols, basic self-care activities, such as grooming, oral hygiene, dressing, and eating, are used as guidelines to determine the functional capacity of the post–myocardial infarction patient. Impairments are usually related to a lack of physical endurance. *Conditions in Occupational Therapy: Effect on Occupational Performance* by Hansen and Atchinson

71. a. An initial spinal cord lesion results in spinal shock, which lasts for 1 week to 3 months. During spinal shock, the spinal cord may function as though it is alive both above and below the level. The problem is one of communication; the brain cannot receive sensory information beyond the lesion site and cannot volitionally control motor function below that point (p. 187–188). Eventually, this subsides, and in upper motor neuron lesion, spasticity normally increases. *Conditions in Occupational Therapy: Effect on Occupational Performance* by Hansen and Atchinson

72. c. With diabetes, sensorimotor function is influenced by the development of peripheral neuropathy. Peripheral neuropathy may result in diminished to absent tactile processing. Tactile issues may result in fine and gross motor incoordination and eventually muscle atrophy and diminished strength, particularly in the distal extremities. *Conditions in Occupational Therapy: Effect on Occupational Performance* by Hansen and Atchinson

73. d. The most obvious method to obtain information about desired or needed performance is to ask the patient or client. Therefore, to assess self-perception of performance and satisfaction of daily occupations, a semi-structured interview would be helpful. For example, the Canadian Occupational Performance Measure (COPM) and the Occupational Performance History Interview II (OPH II) are instruments used to determine wants and needs related to occupational performance. *Occupational Therapy: Performance, Participation, and Well-Being* by Christiansen and Baum

74. a. Skilled observation entails using professional skills and judgment to watch performance in the actual contexts of interest and making hypotheses about the meaning of those observations to meet the needs of the individuals. *Occupational Therapy: Performance, Participation, and Well-Being* by Christiansen and Baum

75. b. In criterion-referenced measurements, the results are compared to some standard of performance, such as with developmental milestones. *Occupational Therapy: Performance, Participation, and Well-Being* by Christiansen and Baum

76. a. Gravity-eliminated position for testing elbow extension starts with the patient in sitting and the humerus supported at 90 degrees; the elbow is also flexed. The patient is instructed to straighten the elbow while the tester palpates the triceps muscle. *Occupational Therapy for Physical Dysfunction* by Trombly and Radomski

77. b. Stereognosis is a test that supports occupational functioning, such as using the hand to identify common objects. When testing stereognosis, vision is occluded. *Occupational Therapy for Physical Dysfunction* by Trombly and Radomski

78. c. Posttraumatic agitation may include verbalizations and inappropriate sexual behavior but are not seen in all cases of agitation. Increased initiation to task is inconsistent with traumatic brain injury. *Occupational Therapy for Physical Dysfunction* by Trombly and Radomski

79. d. Self-care performance would give the most valid and valuable information in this case. The standard manual muscle test would be contraindicated for someone with abnormal tone and AROM, and sensation can be better assessed through observation of skills as opposed to individual evaluations in these areas. *Stroke Rehabilitation: A Functional-Based Approach* by Gillen and Burkhardt

80. a. Clients with ideational apraxia have difficulty using items in the appropriate ways because of a loss of understanding of the act itself. *Vision, Perception and Cognition* by Zoltan

81. a. Tone that presents with only minimal resistance and the ability to complete full ROM would classify as mild. *Stroke Rehabilitation: A Functional-Based Approach* by Gillen and Burkhardt

82. a. The use of these activities will give you the most information about the client's ability to scan the environment and a tabletop surface. *Vision, Perception and Cognition* by Zoltan

83. c. Clients with body neglect frequently dress only one side of the body, neglecting the affected side. *Vision, Perception and Cognition* by Zoltan

84. c. Ideational apraxia is defined by Zoltan as a disability in carrying out complex sequential motor acts, which is caused by a disruption of the conception, rather than the execution of the motor act. *Vision, Perception and Cognition* by Zoltan

85. c. Hemianopsia results in a loss of vision in one-half of the visual field of an eye, usually on the same side as the lesion. *Occupational Therapy for Physical Dysfunction* by Trombly and Radomski

86. a. A child with a hyporesponsive system will engage in a variety of activities to increase the level of stimulation. *Occupational Therapy for Children* by Case-Smith

87. a. Although all of these may make letter recognition difficult, a weakness with form constancy will make this the most difficult. *Occupational Therapy for Children* by Case-Smith

88. d. Oculomotor control, visual fields, and visual acuity are considered to be primary visual skills and serve as a foundation for the hierarchy of visual perceptual skills. *Occupational Therapy for Children* by Case-Smith

89. c. This will allow the OT to achieve an integrated picture of the child and help to eliminate a problem that may have been overlooked in addition to the handwriting difficulties. *Occupational Therapy for Children* by Case-Smith

90. b. The line of vision dictates head and neck posture. If the screen is too low or too far away from the face, the user must flex the neck and trunk. If the head is held forward, cervical muscles become fatigued. *Ergonomics for Therapists,* 2nd ed. by Jacobs

91. c. Direct pressure over a nerve can cause nerve compression that may lead to a neuropathy. Accompanying symptoms may be muscle weakness, numbness, and tingling over the distribution area of the nerve. *Ergonomics for Therapists,* 2nd ed. by Jacobs

92. c. The inability to adjust the screen height leads to more neck flexion because of the forward head posture. This can cause neck and shoulder pain. *Ergonomics for Therapists,* 2nd ed. by Jacobs

93. b. The most efficient work space is a 10-inch square directly in front of the worker. *Ergonomics for Therapists,* 2nd ed. by Jacobs

94. d. Maximum floor to high forward reach for an average American adult in a wheelchair is 53½ inches. *Ergonomics for Therapists,* 2nd ed. by Jacobs

95. d. The turning radius for a wheelchair to do a 360-degree turn is 74 inches square. *Ergonomics for Therapists,* 2nd ed. by Jacobs

96. b. In this case, function is returning and the primary issue related to the presence of edema. The therapist should be concerned with preventing further complications that could accompany swelling, such as loss of range of motion. *Introduction to Splinting: A Clinical Reasoning & Problem Solving Process* by Coppard and Lohman

97. c. Cruising is the shifting of weight onto one leg and stepping to the side with the other. *Occupational Therapy for Children* by Case-Smith

98. d. PDD is characterized by impairment in communication and severe impairment in reciprocal social relationships. *Psychosocial Occupational Therapy* by Cara and MacRae

99. c. In spastic diplegia, the term diplegia identifies the parts of the body that are affected by the spasticity. Diplegia refers to involvement of two extremities or identical parts of both sides of the body. *Occupational Therapy for Children* by Case-Smith

100. d. Ataxia is characterized by a wide-based gait and difficulty shifting weight in motion, which results in unsteady ambulation. *Occupational Therapy for Physical Dysfunction* by Trombly and Radomski

101. d. The purpose of the screening process is to determine the need for further evaluation. Screening includes reviewing relevant information before the formal evaluation. *Occupational Therapy for Physical Dysfunction* by Trombly and Radomski

102. a. Visual-motor tasks generally involve replicating visual stimuli through motor output, such as writing or drawing. *Occupational Therapy for Children* by Case-Smith

103. b. Rocking while positioned on the hands and knees is consistent with the motor development of an 8-month-old. *Occupational Therapy for Children* by Case-Smith

104. b. The spinal deformity in the upper back (thoracic region) curvature has a convexity posterior known as kyphosis. *Occupational Therapy for Children* by Case-Smith

105. b. Developmental disability is manifested before the person becomes 22 years old and results in substantial functional limitations in a major life activity. *Occupational Therapy Principles and Practice* by Punwar and Peloquin

106. a. Children who are autistic often exhibit problems in many areas, but the most pronounced area of impairment is usually in socialization. *Occupational Therapy Performance, Participation, and Well-being* by Christiansen and Baum

107. c. Oscillopsia or oscillating vision is a condition where objects seem to move backward and forward, wiggle, or jerk. When assessing movement in an individual with this condition, it is important to determine if there are any balance issues by assessing equilibrium during standing and with movement, as well as spatial orientation. *Quick Reference to Occupational Therapy* by Reed

108. d. An elderly person may become suspicious of what is being said and experience fear of being talked about; this is a paranoid response. *Psychosocial Occupational Therapy* by Cara and MacRae

109. a. Using a slower gait can conserve energy, thereby preventing muscle fatigue. *Psychosocial Occupational Therapy* by Cara and MacRae

110. c. Automatic postural stabilization involves a combination of three sensory system including the use of vision, somatosensory (proprioception), and vestibular input. *Functional Performance in Older Adults* by Bonder and Wagner

111. c. The presence of a throw rug could result in a fall, which would be far more hazardous to the health of an elderly client than the other objects in the environment. In the elderly, falls are

the major cause of fractures. *Functional Performance in Older Adults* by Bonder and Wagner

112. d. Psychological age includes self-esteem, learning, memory, and perception; these are all psychological functions. *Functional Performance in Older Adults* by Bonder and Wagner

113. b. Generally if other pathology is not present, the underlying reason for an elderly person to use the wall for stability is because of poor balance or postural control, which is a central nervous system function. *Functional Performance in Older Adults* by Bonder and Wagner

114. b. The frail elderly require assistance for functional tasks because of client factors that impede living independently. *Functional Performance in Older Adults* by Bonder and Wagner

115. d. Family structures are dynamic because they change through births, deaths, and marriage. *Functional Performance in Older Adults* by Bonder and Wagner

116. b. In the elderly, there is research that suggest that tactile sensation decreases with aging along with related sense of kinesthesia, which is awareness of the body in space. *Aging: The Health Care Challenge* by Lewis

117. d. Impairment is a loss or abnormality of function at the body system or organ level, which may or may not be permanent, and there may or may not be a resultant disability/handicap/dysfunction. *Ergonomics for Therapists,* by Jacobs

118. d. According to the *OT Practice Framework* (AOTA, 2002), the process of service delivery as applied within the profession's domain includes evaluation, intervention, and outcomes assessment.

119. c. To be effective, occupational therapy's contribution to the transition process must focus on the student's future: What does the student want to do or expect to do? What environments does the student use now, and what environments will they use in the future? How will the student's current interests and abilities mesh with future roles and activities? Effective transition services facilitate students' engagement in meaningful work roles, community and recreational participation, and ongoing positive social relationships. *Work Principles and Practice. Self-Paced Clinical Course* by AOTA

120. a. An employer may not make a preemployment inquiry on an application form or in an interview regarding whether or to what extent a person has a disability or medical condition and if he or she requires reasonable accommodation. The employer may ask a job applicant whether they can perform particular job functions. *Ergonomics and the Management of Musculoskeletal Disorders* by Sanders

121. b. It is most probable that the cervical disc herniation at C6 is causing weakness in the C6 dermatome and myotome of the right upper extremity. *Ergonomics and the Management of Musculoskeletal Disorders* by Sanders

122. a. Specific upper-extremity MSDs recognized by the International Classification of Diseases include lateral epicondylitis, but does not include primary osteoarthritis, Dupuytren's contractures, or cervical stenosis. *Ergonomics and the Management of Musculoskeletal Disorders* by Sanders

123. d. Work-related MSDs are a multifactorial problem meaning that both work- and non–work-related risk factors contribute to the process. Diabetes, obesity, and a sedentary lifestyle would be considered medical or non–work-related risk factors rather than a work-related risk factor. *Ergonomics and the Management of Musculoskeletal Disorders* by Sanders

124. d. The duration of activity performance or the amount of time it takes to complete an activity is a measure of efficiency. Less time means more efficient; more time means less efficient. *Williard & Spackman's Occupational Therapy,* 10th ed. by Crepeau, Cohn, and Schell

125. c. According the *OT Practice Framework* (AOTA, 2002), political and cultural context of the work environment would include issues such as administration and management of an organization, the employees, and the organizational culture. *Work Program Practice: Aiming for Successful Context Management* by Alexander

126. b. According the *OT Practice Framework* (AOTA, 2002), activity demands include objects used, such as tools (i.e., screwdriver) and required actions (i.e., the skill required to utilize a screwdriver).

127. d. Through assessment of the workstation, the OT is analyzing the client's occupational performance. This involves understanding

the demands of the activity, the range of skills involved in performing the activity, and the various cultural means that might be ascribed to the activity. *Willard & Spackman's Occupational Therapy*, 10th ed. by Crepeau, Cohn, and Schell

128. a. FCEs can serve many functions. However, determining if impairments exist is essentially diagnosing a client, which is beyond the scope of occupational therapy practice. Only medical doctors are qualified to determine impairments. *Guides to the Evaluation of Permanent Impairment,* 2nd ed. by the American Medical Association, and *Ergonomics and the Management of Musculoskeletal Disorders* by Sanders

129. d. According to the *OT Practice Framework* (AOTA, 2002), strength and effort pertains to skills that require generation of muscle force appropriate for effective interaction with task objects including moving, transporting, and lifting.

130. a. According to the *OT Practice Framework* (AOTA, 2002), information exchange refers to giving and receiving information within an occupation including asking, engaging, and sharing.

131. d. de Quervain's disease affects the abductor pollicis longus (APL) and extensor pollicis brevis (EPB) within the first dorsal compartment of the wrist. Finklestein's test stretches the tendons (APL, EPB) in the first dorsal compartment. *Ergonomics and the Management of Musculoskeletal Disorders* by Sanders

132. d. According to the *OT Practice Framework* (AOTA, 2002), cultural context includes political issues and aspects, such as laws and statues.

133. a. Prolonged exposure to vibration from vibrating power hand tools has been known to affect workers' overall health and to contribute to flexor tenosynovitis and carpal tunnel syndrome. *Ergonomics and the Management of Musculoskeletal Disorders* by Sanders

134. c. Sensory modulation is dependent on an individual's ability to filter sensations and attend to those that are relevant. A child who has difficulty modulating auditory input may have difficulty filtering out background noise and attending to the lesson that is being presented. *Sensory Integration: Theory and Practice* by Bundy

135. d.   The OT would likely choose an evaluation that measures the child's ability to participate in self-care, mobility, and social functions. One example of such an assessment is the Pediatric Evaluation of Disability Inventory (PEDI). It was designed to measure functional independence in children 6 months to 7½ years of age; however, it may also be used with children who have significant limitations. *Occupational Therapy for Children* by Case-Smith

136. a.   Given the child's age and diagnosis, as well as the treatment setting, the OT would likely choose an assessment that measure gross and fine motor skills. An evaluation such as the Bruininks–Oseretsky Test of Motor Performance measures both fine and gross motor skills. *Occupational Therapy for Children* by Case-Smith

137. a.   Hand skill development is dependent on vision. As early as infancy, children begin to look around them and reach toward items that entice them visually. As they further develop, children start to adjust their hands in response to characteristics, sizes, and shapes of objects. Providing intervention in a well-lit room will allow the child to use his or her visual skills to the fullest extent to guide motor movements. *Occupational Therapy for Children* by Case-Smith

138. d.   All of the reflexive behaviors influence grasp. However, a persistent grasp reflex can interfere with a child's ability to release objects. The presence of the avoiding reaction actually supports the release of an object. *Hand Function in the Child* by Henderson and Pehoski

139. c.   Strabismus is a visual impairment that causes an inability of the eyes to converge properly on an image. As a result, both eyes may not be directed at the same point. This condition is cause by muscle imbalance and often results in double vision. *Occupational Therapy for Children* by Case-Smith

140. c.   Aversive response to movement is a type of sensory modulation dysfunction characterized by the autonomic nervous system's reactions to movements that most individuals would consider non-noxious; it is thought to be the result of poor processing of vestibular information. *Sensory Integration: Theory and Practice* by Bundy

141. a.   Frequent negative behaviors, such as screaming, crying, withdrawing, or aggression, in response to age-appropriate activities, suggests sensory defensiveness. Sensory defensiveness

is suspected in infants or young children when a consistent pattern of aversive responses are observed during daily activities. *Pediatric Occupational Therapy and Early Intervention* by Case-Smith

142. d.   A continuous intrathecal baclofen pump is a medical intervention used to control spasticity. It is typical for a physician to request static splints after the insertion of the pump to provide the client with a constant stretch and further limit the effects of spasticity. The function of a shunt is to reduce the pressure in the brain caused by hydrocephalus. *Occupational Therapy for Children* by Case-Smith

143. c.   Children who have brachial plexus lesions often hold the affected extremity in a characteristic posture, with shoulder adducted and internally rotated, elbow extended, forearm pronated, and wrist flexed. In addition, their hands may be weak, and wasting of the small hand muscles may be evident. *Occupational Therapy for Children* by Case-Smith

144. b.   The sequence of self-care acquisition is largely dependent on perceptual abilities, particularly in terms of dressing. A higher level of perceptual abilities is required to button a shirt than unbutton one. To button a shirt the child must be able to line up the buttons and the buttonholes, whereas in unbuttoning the child just has to push the button through the hole. Both unbuttoning and buttoning require a similar degree of strength. *Hand Function in the Child* by Henderson and Pehoski

145. b.   Alignment or baseline orientation refers to the placement of text on and within the writing guidelines. Letter formation involves five features: improper letter forms, poor leading in and out of letters, incomplete closure of letters, and incorrect ascenders and descenders. Spacing includes the dispersion of letters within words and words within sentences along with text organization on the entire sheet of paper. Near-point copying is producing letters or words from a nearby model, commonly on the same page or on the same horizontal surface. *Occupational Therapy for Children* by Case-Smith

146. a.   The Sensory Profile provides the OT with a platform for theory-based decision making and renders salient information regarding a child's sensory processing abilities and how these abilities impact functional performance in typical activities of daily living. *Sensory Integration: Theory and Practice* by Bundy

147. c. A lower set thumb may decrease the functional opposition skills of a child with Down syndrome. *Hand Function in the Child* by Henderson and Pehoski

148. c. Short-term visual memory is the ability to hold information received through the visual channel for approximately 30 seconds. A student who has difficulty copying from the board because they cannot remember what word to write down next may have difficulty with visual memory. *Occupational Therapy for Children* by Case-Smith

149. a. Aversive responses to vestibular input include nausea, vomiting, dizziness, vertigo, excessive emotional reactions, and other symptoms associated with autonomic nervous system functioning. *Sensory Integration: Theory and Practice* by Bundy

150. d. The child would most likely have difficulty catching a ball because the visual system plays a major role in anticipating the location of moving objects and guiding movements to these locations. *Sensory Integration: Theory and Practice* by Bundy

151. c. Neuromaturation theories assume that child development is hierarchical and that skills increase based on functional changes related to client factors. *Occupational Therapy for Children* by Case-Smith

152. c. Diplegia refers to mild involvement in upper extremities and significant involvement in lower extremities. Involvement in all four extremities would be considered quadriplegia or tetraplegia. Hemiplegia refers to involvement in both the upper and lower extremities on one side of the body. *Occupational Therapy for Children* by Case-Smith

153. c. Norm-referenced assessments allow the occupational therapist to compare a client's score to the normative group or the population that the assessment's psychometric properties are based on. Because of their psychometric properties, norm-referenced tests yield average scores, standard scores, percentile ranks, and age equivalences. *Occupational Therapy for Children* by Case-Smith

154. d. To calculate for adjusted age, the chronological age must first be determined. In this case the child is 6 months old, or 24 weeks. Next, subtract the actual birth date from the due date to determine the prematurity value. In this case, the prematurity value is 10 weeks. Finally, subtract the prematurity value from

the chronological age to determine the adjusted age. In this example, the adjusted age is 14 weeks or 3½ months. Adjusted age is only used for the first 2 years of life. *Occupational Therapy for Children* by Case-Smith

155. c. Both unscrewing a bottle top and picking up a pencil involve simple rotation skills because the fingers move as a unit to partially turn the object. Activities to work on simple rotation are often presented to the child while their forearm is pronated. *Hand Function in the Child* by Henderson and Pehoski

156. c. According to typical development, a child should be able to begin to stand without support between 10–13 months of age. Walking with support typically only emerges around 13 months, and bending down to pick up a toy without external support begins to emerge around 19 months. *Occupational Therapy in Children* by Case-Smith

157. d. Children that demonstrate gravitational insecurity typically become upset when their heads are tipped back or their feet are taken off of the ground. This dysfunction is most closely related to the vestibular system. *Sensory Integration: Theory and Practice* by Bundy

158. a. A top-down assessment approach first looks at the child's occupational profile, which may include how the child participates at school. After the OT examines occupational participation, the OT may decide that information is needed to better understand the impact of the child's personal factors in relation to occupation. In this case, the OT would then proceed to further evaluate the child's skills and client factors. *Occupational Therapy in Children* by Case-Smith

159. c. Several models provide insight into the person-environment-occupation relationship. A primary difference between MOHO and other models that consider this relationship is the concept of volition. According to Kielhofner, volition is a "collection of dispositions and self knowledge that enables persons to anticipate, choose, experience, and interpret their occupational behavior (p. 39)." *Occupational Therapy in Children* by Case-Smith and *A Model of Human Occupation: Theory & Application* by Kielhofner

160. d. Tongue thrust, an in-and-out movement pattern, is frequently seen in association with increased extensor tone. This movement pattern may also develop to compensate for tongue retraction. The persistence of tongue thrust inhibits the development of

more refined movements necessary for feeding. *Handling the Young Child with Cerebral Palsy at Home* by Finnie

161. b. A clear hand preference within the first year of life may be indicative of central nervous system dysfunction or an upper motor neuron disorder. *Pediatric Occupational Therapy and Early Intervention* by Case-Smith

162. d. Only holding paper with one hand and using scissors to cut with the opposite hand would address bilateral integration skills. Weight shifting in preparation to kick a ball would address postural adaptations; swiping at a balloon with either hand and throwing a tennis ball at a target would address motor planning and visual-motor integration skills. *Pediatric Occupational Therapy and Early Intervention* by Case-Smith

163. a. The dynamic tripod grasp is an ergonomically effective method to hold a utensil for the purpose of writing. When using a dynamic tripod grasp, the individual's web space is open, and the thumb, index, and middle fingers make the most efficient strokes. *Occupational Therapy for Children* by Case-Smith

164. a. Motor planning, or praxis, is comprised three components: ideation (deciding to complete an action), planning (developing a motor plan or sequence of actions), and execution (completing motor movements to carry out the plan or sequence of actions). *Sensory Integration: Theory and Practice* by Bundy

165. d. Out of all of the senses, the tactile, proprioceptive, and vestibular senses are considered the most salient in terms of the development of adaptive responses. *Sensory Integration: Theory and Practice* by Bundy

166. d. A child who repeatedly climbs on to the top of the monkey bars and jumps off may be seeking both vestibular and proprioceptive input. The child would gain vestibular input while falling through the air; he would gain proprioceptive input while using his arms and legs to climb up the to the top of the monkey bars and while landing on his feet. *Sensory Integration: Theory and Practice* by Bundy

167. b. The Barthel index measures basic ADL functioning, which we have established as independent. The Functional Independence Measure primarily measures basic ADL functioning as well. The Functional Test for the Hemiparetic Upper Extremity will only capture the patient's motor control ability in their weak arm. The Kohlman Evaluation of Living Skills rates 17 tasks

including safety awareness, money management, and phone book usage needed to live independently. *Occupational Therapy Practice Skills for Physical Dysfunction* by Pedretti and Early

168. b. Clonus is a form of spasticity characterized by repetitive contractions in the antagonistic muscles. Synergy is a description of the muscles that contract in a typical sequence with hypertonicity. Spinal hypertonia describes increased muscle tone from a spinal cord injury. Flaccidity is the absence of muscle tone. *Occupational Therapy Practice Skills for Physical Dysfunction* by Pedretti and Early

169. a. Ataxia is difficulty with movement in relation to range, force, and regularity. This is a cerebellar disorder. Chorea differs from ataxia in that there are purposeless, involuntary, jerky movements. Athetoid movements are described as continuous, slow, arrhythmic movements. *Occupational Therapy Practice Skills for Physical Dysfunction* by Pedretti and Early

170. d. A visual history is important so that any premorbid issues may be integrated into the evaluation. The patient may have worn glasses for decreased acuity or have conditions that previously affected oculomotor control. *Occupational Therapy Practice Skills for Physical Dysfunction* by Pedretti and Early

171. a. The positioning described is a synergy pattern that indicates spasticity. The Ashworth assesses muscle tone. The Jebsen and Wolf evaluate specific hand function. The MMT assesses muscle strength. *Occupational Therapy Practice Skills for Physical Dysfunction* by Pedretti and Early

172. c. Rigidity is an increase of muscle tone of agonist and antagonist muscles simultaneously. Both groups of muscles contract steadily, leading to increased resistance to passive movement in any direction throughout the ROM. Hypertonus and spasticity describe a type of increased muscle tone with spasticity being velocity-dependent. Clonus is a repetitive response to a stimulus on the muscle. *Occupational Therapy Practice Skills for Physical Dysfunction* by Pedretti and Early

173. a. Visual inattention will create asymmetry in functional tasks that a person performs. A right field cut would possibly have been demonstrated if the food had been missed on the right side. A confrontation evaluation would be needed to assess oculomotor control. Diplopia may be present but an interview and assessment would be needed in this situation. *Occupational*

Therapy Practice Skills for Physical Dysfunction by Pedretti and Early

174. d. Forgetting to turn off the water would be an example of impaired attention to task. Verbal cues to put the toothbrush into the patient's mouth may indicate difficulty with sequencing or motor control. Verbal cues to put toothpaste on the brush before brushing the patient's teeth could be a sequencing difficulty. Assistance for positioning the toothbrush under the faucet is the best choice in describing a spatial relations difficulty of judging distances, distinguishing one form from another. *Vision, Perception and Cognition* by Zoltan

175. b. Clonus is a form of spasticity characterized by repetitive contractions in the antagonistic muscles caused by hypertonus, which may occur because of upper or lower motor neuron dysfunction. Aphasia, agnosia, and apraxia are all upper motor neuron deficits. *Occupational Therapy Practice Skills for Physical Dysfunction* by Pedretti and Early

176. a. If acuity cannot be corrected, you may be able to compensate for the deficit by increasing the font size, contrast, or illumination. If the TV is affecting the evaluation this would be because of attentional impairment, not decreased acuity. Increasing contrast should be a dark color on a light color and not two similar colors together. By reading the questions you will not be able to evaluate the person's ability to read and follow directions. *Vision, Perception and Cognition* by Zoltan

177. d. Aphasia is seen in persons with left hemisphere CVA. Inattention should not be as much of an issue because of the quiet environment. *Occupational Therapy Practice Skills for Physical Dysfunction* by Pedretti and Early

178. c. If soft tissue shortening has occurred over time, low load prolonged stretch splinting would be ideal. This technique is very different than stretching and weight bearing, which typically position the patient into the greatest amount of stretch tolerated. AROM and PROM will have significantly less effect on the structures. *Occupational Therapy Practice Skills for Physical Dysfunction* by Pedretti and Early

179. b. Topographical orientation is the awareness of one's position in relation to the environment. Persons that have topographical disorientation may become confused when leaving a room or building. *Occupational Therapy Practice Skills for Physical Dysfunction* by Pedretti and Early

180. a. Narrative reasoning is a client-centered approach that encourages the individual to share their story, history, concerns, and goals. This approach can assist in understanding habits, routines, roles, and how the illness or condition has affected one's occupational performance, which are all parts of the occupational profile. *Occupational Therapy for Physical Dysfunction* by Trombly and Radomski

181. c. The OT must be aware of the side effects of psychotropic drugs, including dry mouth, tremors, and constipation. In view of the patient's recent change in drugs, it would be highly suspected that these are side effects of the drug. The patient should be referred to the prescribing psychiatrist. This could be a possibility as the primary care physician would evaluate the patient and refer the patient to the psychiatrist if needed. It would be ill-advised to treat the patient symptomatically, because the therapist is aware that these could be the side effects of the drug. *Occupational Therapy for Children* by Case-Smith

182. c. The patient shows traits of obsessive-compulsive disorder in the patient's repetitive and time-consuming cleaning and arranging. The child becomes fretful if the child is unable to do it. ADHD is characterized by significant difficulty with selective and/or sustained attention to tasks. There are no fluctuations in behavior from extreme to moderate to describe bipolar disorder. *Occupational Therapy for Children* by Case-Smith

183. b. PDD is characterized by abnormal sensory processing, and restricted, repetitive, and stereotyped patterns of behavior, interests, and activities. Pervasive long-standing feelings of uneasiness are a prime feature of anxiety disorder, whereas difficulty with selective or sustained attention to tasks is a characteristic of ADHD. *Occupational Therapy for Children* by Case-Smith

184. a. Some newborns endure nursing and medical procedures, such as lung suctioning, intubations, and nasal gastric feeding, wherein hard plastic tubes are inserted in the mouth and throat. These tubes almost always cause gagging and coughing. If the experiences are repeated, the infant develops oral tactile defensiveness to all oral sensory inputs. Lack of oral feedings, oral stimulation, and a lack of exposure to different food textures can also lead to oral hypersensitivity. However, lack of oral experiences may be the easiest type of sensory defensiveness to overcome. Poor nutrition does not necessarily cause oral sensitivity. Respiratory problems could cause

swallowing problems, not oral hypersensitivity. *Occupational Therapy for Children* by Case-Smith

185. d. At 4–5 years of age, the child is independent in toileting. *Occupational Therapy for Children* by Case-Smith

186. a. Children with autism have severe sensory integrative problems. Play in such children is characterized by stereotyped movements or types of play, decreased play organization, and decreased manipulation of toys. Limited and abnormal movement and decreased and lack of opportunities for social play are the play characteristics of children with cerebral palsy. *Occupational Therapy for Children* by Case-Smith

187. a. The features of letter formation that impact legibility are incomplete closure of letters and inadequate rounding of letters. In addition, if the ascenders and descenders are not properly formed, legibility is poor. However, baseline orientation refers to the placement of letters within the writing guidelines and does affect legibility but is not a feature of letter formation. An inconsistent slant too affects legibility, but is not a feature of letter formation. *Occupational Therapy for Children* by Case-Smith

188. c. At 9 months of age a child would experience a strong urge to be upright. The child would be standing and cruising with the support of furniture or people. An infant who is developing typically would reach the locomotion milestone of creeping and moving from sitting to quadruped and back at around 8 months. *Occupational Therapy for Children* by Case-Smith

189. b. The term marginal ambulator is used to describe children who have cerebral palsy with less involvement. These children ambulate but are unable to do so at a reasonable rate of speed or with acceptable endurance. Because they are not capable of producing efficient mobility themselves, they need augmentative mobility provided by the power wheelchair. *Occupational Therapy for Children* by Case-Smith

190. c. The gestational age, which needs to be determined for this child, refers to the total number of weeks the infant was in utero before birth. Determination is based on the last menstrual period, ultrasound results, or a physical examination of the infant. This is useful for determining problems for small infants in utero and postbirth. Postconceptional age refers to the infant's age in relation to conception and is obtained by adding the weeks since birth to the infant's gestational age and is used

until 40–44 weeks. Chronologic age refers to the infant's actual age. Corrected age refers to how old the infant would be if born at term rather than prematurely. *Occupational Therapy for Children* by Case-Smith

191. c.   The irises of a preterm infant do not constrict significantly until about 30–34 weeks. These infants are not able to close their eyelids tightly until 30–34 weeks, so the occupational therapist should help protect the infant's eyes from exposure to bright or direct light. *Occupational Therapy for Children* by Case-Smith

192. b.   Mechanical ventilation is ventilation in which the machine controls or assists breathing by mechanically inflating the lungs. Bag and mask ventilation is used for resuscitation of an infant at delivery, during acute deterioration, or to increase oxygenation after an apneic spell. *Occupational Therapy for Children* by Case-Smith

193. b.   A cataract occurs when the lens of the eye changes from clear to cloudy or opaque. Although it is often the result of heredity, childhood cataracts can be associated with juvenile diabetes. *Occupational Therapy for Children* by Case-Smith

194. b.   A child with myopia, or nearsightedness, sees most clearly at close range and much less efficiently at a distance. The eyeball is too long or refractive power is too strong; therefore, the focus point is in front of the retina. This causes the child to have blurred vision, and external strabismus is possible when the individual is looking at a distance. The child often holds printed material close to the eyes. *Occupational Therapy for Children* by Case-Smith

195. c.   Although visual acuity can be determined by the PL test, it is more useful for assessing visual improvement in children with amblyopia and for detecting differences in vision between the eyes. *Occupational Therapy for Children* by Case-Smith

196. a.   Recurrent otitis media can cause conductive losses that are temporary when detected early and can be corrected by medical or surgical means. *Occupational Therapy for Children* by Case-Smith

197. b.   With a low-frequency loss, vowels are missed but many consonants are heard. Voices sound weak and thin, but they are understandable if close enough to the speaker. *Occupational Therapy for Children* by Case-Smith

198. a. Tourette's is distinct from other tic and anxiety disorders, because it presents with both motor and vocal tics at the same time. *DSM-IV-TR* by the American Psychiatric Association

199. a. Using an holistic view to understand the environment in which older adults function, OTs are specially trained in environmental adaptation that addresses the needs of older adults in areas related to the physical, social, emotional, spiritual, and cognitive contexts. *Psychosocial Occupational Therapy: A Clinical Practice* by Cara and MacRae

200. d. The Adolescent Role Assessment is a tool that evaluates the adolescent's role performance and social functioning. The other tools are either from different frameworks or address the needs of other age groups. *Assessments in Occupational Therapy mental Health: An Integrative Approach* by Hemphill

201. a. The Adolescent Role Assessment is the only tool in the answers that assesses performance during a specific time frame of an individual's lifespan. *Assessments in Occupational Therapy Mental Health: An Integrative Approach* by Hemphill

202. c. Personal feelings must not be allowed to impact the therapeutic relationship and any personal judgment of the client or his or her behavior must be avoided. The focus needs to on nonjudgmental, professional evaluation of the person's occupational performance and functioning. *Assessment in Occupational Therapy Mental Health: An Integrative Approach* by Hemphill

203. a. Giving advice or sending the patient to her doctor to get the decision made is not appropriate therapeutic behavior. The OT's role is to help the patient to review her options and encourage her to make the best decision she can for herself. *Mental Health Concepts and Techniques for the Occupational Therapy Assistant* by Early

204. a. Ethically, it is not appropriate to ignore the comment or judge the patient. Suicidal thoughts are not normal, and sharing such personal information about yourself would create a boundary issue. It is important to find out more about these feelings to determine what action should be taken to keep the patient safe. *Mental Health Concepts and Techniques for the Occupational Therapy Assistant* by Early

205. b. In a behavioral approach the focus is on the behaviors an ineffective learning. Emphasis is placed on the present and

learning new behaviors to replace the ineffective ones. *Group Dynamics in Occupational Therapy* by Cole

206. b. Projective techniques can be used to help a patient gain insight concerning his or her behavior, etc. The patient must be the one to interpret the outcomes of the tasks in which he or she engages, because the patient is the only one that can understand the true attached meanings. *Group Dynamics in Occupational Therapy* by Cole

207. b. Behavior of a healthy person must be within the social boundaries of their environment. Everyone experiences some stress in their lives, but how a person handles that stress will impact their health. Being able to realize your goals is evidence of successful occupational functioning and positive mental health. *Mental Health Concepts and Techniques for the Occupational Therapy Assistant* by Early

208. c. This patient's dysfunction is not caused by faulty learning. Rather it is caused by the lack of exposure to age appropriate learning. Therefore, the Developmental Frame of Reference will best help to guide the OT's decision making in the choice of goals and occupations utilized in treatment. *Group Dynamics in Occupational Therapy* by Cole

209. b. By definition, delirium is a disturbance of consciousness that develops over a short period of time and is not associated with a dementia. It involves a reduced ability to focus, sustain, or shift attention. *DSM-IV-TR* by the American Psychiatric Association

210. d. This condition has a gradual onset and patients gradually decline in functioning. *DSM-IV-TR* by the American Psychiatric Association

211. b. Personality disorders are noted in Axis II of the multiaxial classification system. *DSM-IV-TR* by the American Psychiatric Association

212. b. General medical conditions are found under the Axis III of the multiaxial classification system. *DSM-IV-TR* by the American Psychiatric Association

213. b. Intellectual disabilities are noted under Axis II of the multiaxial classification system. *DSM-IV-TR* by the American Psychiatric Association

214. c. Psychosocial and environmental problems are noted under Axis IV of the multiaxial classification system. *DSM-IV-TR* by the American Psychiatric Association

215. d. Cognitive–behavioral therapy is one of the most frequent approaches used for chronic pain management. Its purpose is to help individuals to understand the dynamics of pain and develop coping skills. Multiple methods are use to assist individuals in understanding the relationship between emotions, thoughts, and the physical body including relaxation therapy, visualization, activity pacing, and assertiveness training. *Psychosocial Occupational Therapy: A Clinical Practice* by Cara and MacRae

216. a. A labile affect is characterized by rapid fluctuations in mood. Manic patients often display such emotional lability. *DSM-IV-TR* by the American Psychiatric Association and *Psychopathology and Function* by Bonder

217. a. Although many patients with depression have decreased motivation and involvement in occupation, the level of inactivity described here for the extended time period is seen in catatonic patients. *Psychopathology and Function* by Bonder

218. c. Manic episodes involve a distinct period of abnormal, elevated, expansive, or irritable mood. Patients with bipolar disorder I experience a manic episode with no major depressive episodes in the past. *Psychosocial Occupational Therapy: A Clinical Practice* by Cara and MacRae

219. a. Flight of ideas involves rapid, constant verbalization with multiple shifts in topics discussed. *Psychopathology and Function* by Bonder

220. d. Patients with this disorder have a need for admiration and are unwilling to recognize or identify with the needs of others. *DSM-IV-TR* by the American Psychiatric Association

221. b. The patient is suffering from depression that is impacting the patient's occupational performance. The symptoms have been of a short duration and are related to the many life changes that would be identified in Axis IV. *DSM-IV-TR* by the American Psychiatric Association

222. b. Patients with conversion disorders can experience deficits in motor and or sensory functioning that suggests a medical condition, but no evidence of a medical cause can be found. Psychological factors are determined to be associated with the

loss of function, involving internal conflicts or stressors. *DSM-IV-TR* by the American Psychiatric Association

223. a. Exposure to a phobic situation invariably provokes an anxiety response that disrupts occupational functioning. The person recognizes that the fear is unreasonable and will try to avoid the distressful situation. *DSM-IV-TR* by the American Psychiatric Association

224. a. This model of practice would best suit your needs, because it would account for the impact of the environment on performance and would provide assessment tools that could evaluate how retirement has impacted role performance. *Psychosocial Occupational Therapy: A Holistic Approach* by Stein and Cutler

225. a. Level 5 patients are able to organize themselves and handle more complex tasks. *Psychosocial Occupational Therapy: A Holistic Approach* by Stein and Cutler

226. c. This assessment tool uses interview and tasks to evaluate knowledge and performance across the following five areas: self-care, safety and health, money management, transportation and telephone, and work and leisure. Data from this test can be helpful in predicting discharge success. *Psychosocial Occupational Therapy: A Clinical Practice* by Cara and MacRae

227. c. This is a serious condition that can develop rapidly, without warning. It is the only one of the answer choices that is directly life-threatening, because it can result in extreme muscle rigidity, hyperthermia, altered consciousness, and autonomic dysregulation. The incidence of this condition increases if multiple antipsychotic medications are used. *Psychopathology and Function* by Bonder

228. c. Assessing cognitive capabilities and abilities verifies hypotheses about patient performance deficits and establishes a baseline from which to measure improvement in function. *Occupational Therapy for Physical Dysfunction* by Trombly and Radomski

229. c. Based on manual muscle testing grading system, a muscle grade of two (2) indicates that the body part moves through the full range in a gravity eliminated position. *Occupational Therapy for Physical Dysfunction* by Trombly and Radomski

230. c. Sensory testing should begin by first establishing an area that tests within normal limits. This allows the patient to become

familiar with the procedures and the examiner to establish a normal sensibility area for a point of reference. *Hand and Upper Extremity Rehabilitation: A Practical Guide* by Burke, Higgins, McClinton, Saunders, and Valdata

231. b. Using a client-centered approach, the initial step to performing a home assessment is to understand the roles and responsibilities that the individual must perform in that environment. This will provide guidance for the OT in assessing the areas and issues that primarily affect the person when they return home. *Occupational Therapy: Practice Skills for Physical Dysfunction* by Pedretti and Early

232. a. According to the social cognitive theory introduced by Bandura, there are two stages in learning: acquisition and performance. During acquisition, a child observes the behavior of others and determines the consequences, and these observations are stored in memory for later use. *Occupational Therapy for Children* by Case-Smith

233. c. Practitioners should first determine the extent to which individuals with TBI can scan, attend, follow, and retain directions to interpret performance and responses to other assessments. *Occupational Therapy for Physical Dysfunction* by Trombly and Radomski

234. c. Circumferential measurements are easy and quick to perform and offer an alternative to the use of the volumeter. In cases of a burn with open wounds, the best alternative would be circumferential measurements. *Occupational Therapy for Physical Dysfunction* by Trombly and Radomski

235. b. Using a client-centered approach, individuals are allowed to make choices about intervention. The OT should respect the individual's right to refuse professional services or involvement in research or educational activities. *AOTA: Code of Ethics Document*

236. b. Although all of the steps may need to be assessed in a program related to dysphagia, the first step is to examine oral and pharyngeal control, motion, tone, and sensation of the lips and oral structures and the effects of oral reflexes. *Occupational Therapy for Physical Dysfunction* by Trombly and Radomski

237. d. The Phalen sign is used to test for median nerve compression at the wrist. If flexing the wrist for about 60 seconds elicit

numbness and tingling in the hand over the distribution of the median nerve, this is considered a positive Phalen's sign. *Hand and Upper Extremity Rehabilitation* by Burke, Higgins, McClinton, Saunders, and Valdata

238. c.   Follow testing procedures according to the manual is essential to promote greater reliability of the testing results. *Occupational Therapy for Children* by Case-Smith

239. b.   Endurance can be measures in two ways, both dynamically and statically. Dynamic assessments include: (1) recording the number of repetition of an activity per unit of time; (2) the percent of maximal heart rate during an aerobic activity; and (3) using metabolic equivalent table (MET) level. An example of a static measure is recording the amount of time a contraction is held. *Occupational Therapy Practice Skills for Physical Dysfunction* by Pedretti and Early

240. c.   Reliability is a measure of consistency of the test instrument. The reliability is considered high when two individuals administer the same test and achieve the same results provided that there is no change in the person's status. *Clinical Research in Occupational Therapy* by Stein and Cutler

241. c.   Instruments such as the disk-criminator and aesthesiometer are used to test moving two-point discrimination. Testing begins with the instrument at 5–8 mm distance and is moved randomly and parallel to the long axis of the bone to test the fingers. *Occupational Therapy for Physical Dysfunction* by Trombly and Radomski

242. a.   Kinesthesia refers to perception of position in space. Normally, the stimulus is to place the body part that is being tested on a lateral surface and move in different planes. The person's response is to identify which direction the body part moves, e.g., up and down. *Occupational Therapy for Physical Dysfunction* by Trombly and Radomski

243. b.   Graphesthesia refers to the ability to identify numbers and letters traced on the skin. *Occupational Therapy Practice Skills for Physical Dysfunction* by Pedretti and Early

244. c.   Children with mild spastic diplegia generally have postural insecurity. Children typically react with anxiety and fear when faced with tasks that involves movement in space such as climbing and tend to avoid stairs, escalators, or elevators; moving or high pieces of playground equipment; and uneven surfaces. *Occupational Therapy for Children* by Case-Smith

245. a.   This child may be having visual memory difficulties. Visual memory difficulties present problems when addition and subtraction problems require multiple steps. Children with visual–spatial problems have difficulty in correctly aligning the columns for math problems. Therefore, the difficulties exist because of alignment and not because of calculation skills. *Occupational Therapy for Children* by Case-Smith

246. d.   A stable posture facilitates good directional or controlled reaching. An understanding of postural adaptation is the first issue one must comprehend in relation to reaching. A stable base of support serves as a prerequisite to maximizing functional reach and use of the extremities. *Occupational Therapy Practice Skills for Physical Dysfunction* by Pedretti and Early

247. b.   The next step is to administer a functional motion assessment. Scientific reasoning refers to logical thinking about the patient problem and the occupational therapy process. The logical process parallels scientific inquiry. Two forms of scientific inquiry are used: diagnostic reasoning, which is concerned with understanding the clinical problem, and procedural reasoning, which provides guidance for the sequential steps to follow from the initial referral of the patient to occupational therapy to the discharge or transition to other services. *Willard & Spackman's Occupational Therapy*, 10th ed. by Crepeau, Cohn, and Schell

248. b.   Test-retest reliability is a measurement of the stability of a test over time. Test-retest reliability is proven by giving the test to the same individual on two different occasions. *Clinical Research in Occupational Therapy* by Stein and Cutler

249. a.   Transferring in and out of the bathtub/shower is a functional task that requires weight shifting, thus dynamic balance can be observed. This method of clinical observation employs a method similar to a functional motional assessment. A functional motion assessment is a means of assessing strength, ROM, and motor control by clinically observing the performance or completion of a task. *Occupational Therapy Practice Skills for Physical Dysfunction* by Pedretti and Early

250. d.   Principles of joint protection encourage the use of stronger and larger joints to handle greater forces and loads. For example, use the hips and knees to lift or push and pull item instead of carrying. *Occupational Therapy for Physical Dysfunction* by Trombly and Radomski

251. a.   Norm-referenced tests are standardized and based on the normal populations. When a norm-referenced test is administered, the scores that are collected are compared to the population for which the norms were established. *Clinical Research in Occupational Therapy* by Stein and Cutler

252. a.   Because of a lack of or decreased level of oxygen, persons in advanced stages of COPD may experience confusion and impaired judgment. *Quick Reference in Occupational Therapy* by Reed

253. d.   A functional motion assessment is a means of assessing strength, ROM, and motor control by clinically observing the performance or completion of a task. It can provide clues and allows the OT to observe and assess performance of functional tasks or activities, including compensation. *Occupational Therapy Practice Skills for Physical Dysfunction* by Pedretti and Early

254. a.   Individuals with HIV/AIDS may express shock at the diagnosis and go through the conventional stages of mourning, including any combination of shock and alarm, denial, anger, guilt or fear, altruism, feeling of loss, depression, acceptance, and resignation. *Quick Reference to Occupational Therapy* by Reed

255. b.   Agnosia is a neuropsychological deficit that affects a person's ability to identify objects or people. It is caused by the impairment or loss of processing and interpretation skills related to tactile and visual characteristics. *Quick Reference to Occupational Therapy* by Reed

256. d.   The presence of edema can affect strapping choice on a splint. Circumferential wrapping like Coban or an ace wrap applied to impart even pressure are the preferred choice when splinting a person who has an edematous limb. *Introduction to Splinting: A Clinical Reasoning and Problem Solving Approach* by Coppard and Lohman

257. c.   Physical issues are listed under Axis III. *DSM-IV-TR* by the American Psychiatric Association

258. b.   The ACL test would be the best evaluation to address cognitive issues of memory and recall. The information from this test is helpful in structuring the environment and interactions to best compensate for cognitive limitations. *Mental Health Concepts and Techniques for the Occupational Therapy Assistant* by Early

259. b. To effectively analyze the problem and deal with it in the most effective manner, an OT must first know what the problem is. It is crucial that the history of the patient be examined to help correctly identify what is going on and then determine how you might intervene in the most appropriate way. *Mental Health Concepts and Techniques for the Occupational Therapy Assistant* by Early

260. b. Sharing of information about the patient's hospitalization is up to the patient. The patient has the right to share only what the patient desires. As an adult, the patient may not even want her parents to know about the hospitalization. The OT is responsible for maintaining the patient's confidentiality at all times. *Mental Health Concepts and Techniques for the Occupational Therapy Assistant* by Early

261. a. To improve memory, an initial strategy is to recite the name of items over and over. After this is mastered, the next progressive strategy is to group the same items into categories to see how they might be associated. *Group Dynamics in Occupational Therapy* by Cole

262. b. The symptoms described point to Alzheimer's. No history of substance use was noted and the onset was gradual, not sudden like a head injury. Other symptoms of major depression are not present. *DSM-IV-TR* by the American Psychiatric Association

263. c. For a dual diagnosis the patient must have a substance abuse problem and a psychiatric diagnosis. *Mental Health Concepts and Techniques for the Occupational Therapy Assistant* by Early

264. a. Korsakoff's syndrome is a kind of amnestic condition resulting from long-term alcohol use that involves a person being able to remember things only up to a certain point in his or her life and nothing further. Individuals with Korsakoff's will then often begin to confabulate to fill in the gaps in memory. *Pathology and Function* by Bonder

265. a. Trichotillomania is a condition that causes someone to pull out his or her own hair. *Pathology and Function* by Bonder

266. c. The lower the score on the COTE, the higher the functioning of the patient and the less occupational therapy intervention necessary. It is a comprehensive assessment tool not focused on only memory of motor performance. *Mental Health*

Concepts and Techniques for the Occupational Therapy Assistant by Early

267. b. Relaxation training is a useful and effective intervention to help decrease anxiety disorders and as a means of coping with stress. *Psychosocial Occupational Therapy: A Clinical Practice* by Cara and MacRae

268. b. The patient's thoughts are "flying" from one topic to another. *Psychopathology and Function* by Bonder

269. c. This condition can result in numerous hospitalizations and unnecessary surgeries. *Psychopathology and Function* by Bonder

270. a. These treatments remain controversial but have helped many patients with depression to function more effectively in normal daily occupations. *Conditions in Occupational Therapy: Effect on Occupational Performance* by Hansen

271. b. Polydipsia is a condition involving excessive thirst. Patients with the described behaviors are at risk for drowning themselves. *Conditions in Occupational Therapy: Effect on Occupational Performance* by Hansen

272. b. Individuals who are classified as profoundly mentally handicapped have an IQ of less than 20–25 and function like an infant. They require total supervision and assistance and have very limited communication capabilities. *Conditions in Occupational Therapy: Effect on Occupational Performance* by Hansen

273. d. As a holistic practice, OTs should always be addressing the psychosocial needs of their patients. Once the comatose patient regained consciousness any psychosocial issues would then become a part of the occupational therapy plan for intervention. *Conditions in Occupational Therapy: Effect on Occupational Performance* by Hansen

274. d. Observing the child writing in a natural setting. Handwriting evaluation includes reviewing classroom work, interviewing team members, reviewing the child's history, observing the child writing in the typical environment, evaluating handwriting performance, and evaluating skills that may be impacting the student's handwriting. *Occupational Therapy for Children* by Case-Smith

275. a.   Sensory modulation is primarily assessed through observation and interview. It may be evidenced by sensory defensiveness, gravitational insecurity, aversive response to movement, or poor registration. *Sensory Integration: Theory and Practice* by Bundy

276. c.   At 6–12 months, play development typically includes mouthing toys, accurate and direct reaching, playing with toys at the midline, banging objects together, and grasping and releasing with the fingertips. Based on developmental play, the next milestone of skills is seen at 12–18 months and includes holding crayons, scribbling, stacking blocks, and using one hand to stabilize while the other manipulates. *Occupational Therapy for Children* by Case-Smith

277. b.   The School Function Assessment is a criterion-referenced evaluation tool that considers students' participation, need for task support, and performance in both physical and cognitive/behavioral areas. *Occupational Therapy for Children* by Case-Smith

278. a.   Children who underrespond to sensory input may require more sensory input to obtain and maintain arousal. Their sensory seeking behavior may appear to be risky or dangerous. *Sensory Integration: Theory and Practice* by Bundy

279. c.   Autism includes diagnostic characteristics in the following areas: socialization, communication, restrictive or repetitive behaviors, and sensory processing *Occupational Therapy for Children* by Case-Smith

280. a.   The Clinical Observations of Neuromotor Performance lists observations to be made in the areas of sensory modulation, posture, bilateral integration and sequencing, somatodyspraxia, and eye movements. *Sensory Integration: Theory and Practice* by Bundy

281. b.   Because this patient does not have upper motor neuron deficits, swallowing should be spared at this time. Of the areas listed, feeding should be addressed because of various devices available that can be attached to the wheelchair to assist the patient with eating, such as mobile arm support or some type of arm suspension device. The other reason is that nutritional support is key in the treatment of ALS, and patients may not ask for help if they are unable to finish feeding themselves a meal and thus lose nutritional support. For the other areas, the patient will need assistance from

caregivers and/or family members. The patient may be able to participate in these tasks, but they will need to be modified. *Occupational Therapy Practice Skills for Physical Dysfunction* by Pedretti and Early

CHAPTER 5

Questions for Intervention Planning

This practice examination section covers the topic area of intervention planning. The questions in this section will relate to specific aspects of the intervention planning process, such as goal writing, documentation, and intervention approaches. The objective of this practice examination section is to target content knowledge on the intervention planning process. Use this practice examination to determine your knowledge level in intervention planning process.

1. A 2-year-old child receives early intervention. The occupational therapist (OT) needs to discuss the child's progress with the parents. The OT needs to remember which of the following when communicating with the child's parents:
   a. Talk and do not allow the parents to discuss their concerns and needs as the OT is the expert
   b. Provide the parents with the information about the child's ability when compared to its peers
   c. Tell the parents that it is too bad that all their needs cannot be met and that is just the way things are
   d. Suggest alternative resources to parents even when their requests cannot be met within the system

2. The OT was asked to design a tenodesis splint for a patient with an incomplete C6 spinal cord injury. Which therapeutic goal would this treatment MOST likely support?
   a. Patient will be able to use the hands to perform grasp and release.
   b. Patient will be independent with manipulation of fasteners.
   c. Patient will assist with self-feeding using adapted equipment.
   d. Patient will be able to put on and remove garment using overhead technique.

3. A patient is referred to occupational therapy for splinting. The goal of splinting is to increase range of motion (ROM) that will eventually allow improvement in fine motor coordination and prehension patterns. Which strategy should the OT use to accomplish this goal?
   a. Apply a dynamic splint for controlled motion
   b. Apply prolonged stretch to the joint and soft tissue
   c. Position the extremity in a functional hand position
   d. Position the extremity in the safe hand or antideformity position

4. An OT is treating a patient with a Colles fracture. The patient's forearm has been immobilized for 3 weeks and will require 4 additional weeks in the cast before the patient can begin functional tasks. An initial focus of treatment should be:
   a. Passive ROM (PROM)
   b. Placement of the extremity in a sling
   c. Movement of the joints surrounding the fracture
   d. To avoid treatment until the cast is removed

5. A patient with chronic obstructive pulmonary disease has achieved independence with minimal supervision and is being discharged. Because the patient has no family, alternate living arrangements are needed. The OT should recommend:
   a. A group resident home
   b. Home health care
   c. An assisted living facility
   d. Partial hospitalization

6. A patient with a hip fracture is discharged to home at supervised status in toileting and transfers. In the home program, the OT would recommend that the caregiver:
   a. Initially perform one to two steps of the activities
   b. Provide verbal cueing and physical cueing 25% of the time
   c. Be available to assist the patient with these activities for safety
   d. Provide verbal cueing and directions throughout the activities

7. An OT is treating a patient with a musculoskeletal degenerative disease. Using conditional reasoning to guide the decision making about intervention, the OT would primarily focus on:
   a. The procedures required to assess the individual's performance
   b. The individual's interests, values, concerns, and level of motivation needed to participate in therapy
   c. The impact of the diagnosis on the environmental, social, and future performance of the individual
   d. The individual's explanation and description of the cause of their disability

8. A patient with reflex sympathetic dystrophy syndrome (RSDS), or complex regional pain syndrome (CRPS), has severe edema and increased pain while performing simple grooming activities such as face washing. The initial care plan should focus on:
   a. Pain management
   b. Using the uninvolved extremity
   c. Gentle mobilization
   d. Light activities, such as brushing teeth

9. The OT is treating a patient with a history of coronary artery disease. During the treatment, the patient complains of recurring angina that increases when performing activities in standing. The MOST appropriate course of action by the OT is to:
   a. Stop treatment and contact the physician
   b. Stop treatment until symptoms subside
   c. Assist patient in taking medication for chest pain
   d. Perform treatment in a sitting position

10. A patient diagnosed with Alzheimer's disease is being discharged to home. In preparing the home program, the OT should primarily emphasize:
    a. Cognitive activities to keep the patient's mind engaged
    b. Use of memory aids throughout the patient's home
    c. Recommendations for support services and adult day care
    d. Education of the caregiver on disease process and strategies

11. An OT is designing a intervention plan that focuses on modification of the behavior of a person with a traumatic brain injury (TBI) who exhibits emotional liability and who has difficulty maintaining employment because of chronic lateness. Which contextual factor should guide the OT in decision making?
    a. Physical
    b. Social
    c. Temporal
    d. Cultural

12. A 45-year-old patient is in the first stage of RSDS or CRPS with the classic signs of hand edema, fear of ROM, and pain in the shoulder and hand of the involved extremity. What is the FIRST priority of treatment?
    a. Reduction of edema
    b. Aggressive PROM
    c. Instruct in self ROM
    d. Perform grip strength test

13. A client with a TBI is attending a work rehabilitation program. The long-term goal is to have the patient resume work at a food processing plant handling the canning process. Overall strength and coordination are good, but the client exhibits occasional angry outbursts with other workers. The occupational therapy program should include:
    a. A program that simulates the procedures for canning
    b. Prework hardening with emphasis on social interactions and work readiness
    c. Recommendations to physician for medication to help impulse control
    d. Recommendation for client to delay therapy until behavior is controlled

14. A patient recently experienced a nerve compress that caused the right dominant hand to become limp. Client factors affected are both sensory and motor, including no active wrist extension or forearm supination. Which activity would be the MOST difficult when attempting to use the right hand?
    a. Putting the arm in the sleeve of a shirt
    b. Using a toothbrush
    c. Donning a shirt overhead
    d. Putting on house slippers

15. A patient with a spinal cord injury at the level of C8 would like to be independent in mobility. Based on the expected functional outcomes, the OT would recommend the following piece(s) of adapted equipment:
    a. Manual wheelchair
    b. A motorized wheelchair
    c. A manual wheelchair and sliding board
    d. A walker and wheelchair

16. The OT makes recommendations to a patient after hip replacement surgery for positioning in a wheelchair. Which set of instructions would adhere to safety precautions?
    a. Keep legs abducted with abductor pillow and affected leg in neutral
    b. Keep legs together by using an adductor strap to prevent external rotation of legs
    c. Sit in a regular wheelchair with feet supported on foot rest
    d. Sit in regular wheelchair with affected leg in full extension

17. A 50-year-old patient with a chronic pain condition is receiving occupational therapy for 2 weeks. The patient's complaints include diminished participation in community activities and socialization

and difficulty with some home management tasks. A primary focus of the occupational therapy intervention plan should be:
a. Management of the pain medication
b. Improving patient means of coping and adapting
c. Elimination of pain to participate in social and community activities
d. Teaching biofeedback techniques

18. An essential element of a pain program that the OT should address with every patient is:
a. Coping mechanisms
b. Cognitive skills
c. Medication management
d. Basic activities of daily living (ADL)

19. A patient with carpal tunnel syndrome has been receiving therapy for 2 weeks. The patient recently developed paraesthesia with radiating pain in the forearm, wrist, and hand. The OT should:
a. Begin desensitization activities
b. Stop therapy until symptoms disappear
c. Begin PROM exercise
d. Provide a splint

20. A 6-year-old child in first grade has difficulty coordinating both hands together. The child tends to neglect the left hand. To provide more proprioceptive input to the left arm and to strengthen it, the OT designs a bilateral activity in which the child wears a 1-pound weight on the left wrist. What type of intervention strategy should the OT use?
a. Grading the functional activity
b. Modifying the school environment
c. Training in developmental sequencing
d. Providing augmented sensory cueing and feedback

21. The OT is working with a child who has some behavioral issues and the child's family as well. What are important cultural contextual factors that need to be considered in therapy?
a. The family's view of disability, discipline, and value of independence
b. The school's view of the child's academic performance
c. The family's view of their fit and status in the community
d. The family's financial status and level of education

22. An OT is working with a 68-year-old retiree. The individual shares that it is important to wake at the same time every day, meet friends for coffee at 9 a.m., watch a favorite TV show at 8 p.m. every night,

and play golf on Saturdays. When designing the treatment plan, the OT should heavily focus on:

a. Purposeful activity
b. Occupational performance
c. Habituation
d. Social skills

23. An office worker experienced an injury that resulted in being confined to a wheelchair. When the worker returned to work, an OT was consulted to assess the worker and make recommendations about reasonable accommodations. The OT's recommendations should address:

a. Accessing the building, the work area, and bathrooms
b. Remodeling the building to accommodate the individual's wheelchair
c. Renting a new office space for the individual
d. Investigating other job possibilities

24. The OT is working with a 2-year-old child. The goal is to encourage age appropriate play activities for development. The OT should recommend activities and toys to encourage:

a. Exploratory and social play
b. Attending to others and the environment
c. Functional or relational play
d. Constructive play

25. At a day camp for children with mental retardation, the OT is planning a group activity to work on structured skills, such as being able to follow directions. Although delayed in terms of cognitive maturation, the majority of the children function around a developmental age of 7–8. The OT should select:

a. A puppet show
b. Playground sliding board and swinging
c. Musical chairs
d. A sing-along

26. The OT is designing an intervention plan for a 10-year-old with a learning disability. The intervention plan should focus on developing performance skills related to:

a. Tactile-kinesthetic input
b. Behavioral issues
c. Motor function
d. Cognition

27. A 60-year-old patient with osteoarthritis is receiving home health services. The patient informs the OT about plans to meet friends

for dinner on the upcoming weekend at a local restaurant to try out the adapted eating utensils. Based on the patient's action, the OT should:

a. Meet the patient at the restaurant to ensure proper use of adapted equipment
b. Discharge the patient for occupational therapy services
c. Set more advance goals related to community mobility, such as grocery shopping
d. Advise the patient to wait until other goals are met in therapy

28. While treating a patient with long-standing shoulder joint stiffness, the OT is told by the patient that another OT used heat treatments in the past both before and after functional activities, which was very helpful. Which would be a necessary FIRST step for the OT to take in regard to using physical agent modalities with this patient?

a. Document the length of application and expected response to treatment
b. Position the patient in a comfortable position before applying the treatment
c. Read the patient medical records to confirm the diagnosis
d. Obtain a written prescription from the physician

29. A patient with a brachial plexus injury secondary to an automobile accident has good distal upper extremity function, but the shoulders, elbows, and proximal muscle are weak with a general muscle grade of 3−/5. What piece of adapted equipment may assist this individual in being able to use the extremity for activities, such as feeding and simple grooming of the face and hair?

a. A mobile arm support
b. A forearm splint with a universal cuff
c. A humeral brace
d. A tenodesis splint

30. A patient who sustained a severe heart attack was categorized at a metabolic equivalent table (MET) level of 2–3. The patient has completed the goal of doing homemaking activities, such as washing dishes and ironing. The OT should progress intervention to include the occupational task of:

a. Driving an automobile
b. Performing upper and lower extremity dressing
c. Gardening in the yard
d. Preparing 1–2 meals per day

31. A 30-year-old patient sustained partial thickness burns over a total body surface area of 50% including the patient's bilateral arms and upper trunk. In the acute phase of a burn, the OT should focus on:

    a.   Scar management
    b.   Returning sensation
    c.   Preventing deformity
    d.   Loss of fluid

32.   A patient presents with morning stiffness, joint inflammation, muscle weakness, and difficulty with community mobility and ADLs. The OT's initial goals should be:
    a.   Preservation of muscle strength
    b.   Maintenance of lifestyle
    c.   Relief of pain and inflammation
    d.   Education of patient to use adapted equipment

33.   During a treatment session, the OT observes that the patient can flex the affected shoulder through its full ROM in side lying. The OT should progress to activities that places the extremity in:
    a.   A gravity-assisted position
    b.   A gravity-eliminated position
    c.   A neutral position
    d.   An antigravity position

34.   A patient with peripheral neuropathy has impairment of sensation in bilateral feet and hands. The main focus of treatment should be:
    a.   Desensitization techniques
    b.   Sensory retraining or re-education
    c.   Compensatory techniques related to safety
    d.   Assisting patient in diminishing astereognosis

35.   To evaluate the proper fit of a splint given to a patient, the OT should:
    a.   Instruct the patient to return to the rehab facility if any redness occurs
    b.   Observe for signs of redness after 20 minutes of wearing the splint
    c.   Use a splint pattern to custom make the splint for the patient
    d.   Observe for pressure marks after 24 hours of wearing the splint

36.   An expected outcome for a complete C3 tetraplegic would be:
    a.   The patient will direct a family member or attendant verbally in the patient's care.
    b.   The patient will use a splint for tenodesis action.
    c.   The patient will feed himself with a ratchet splint.
    d.   The patient will assist with dressing.

37. The BEST description of the Model of Human Occupation is:
    a. Activity applies the mechanical principles of kinetics and movement.
    b. Sensorimotor principles are applied to activity and occupation.
    c. Engagement in occupation occurs within the environment.
    d. The central nervous system produces well-modulated movements utilized in occupation.

38. The OT on the spinal cord unit is very frustrated. A 28-year-old patient with C7 tetraplegia refuses to work on dressing techniques, saying that the spouse can assist with dressing. The OT documents that the patient is noncompliant in occupational therapy and will not be able to return to work as an attorney. The occupational therapy supervisor works with the patient one day, and the patient says that the patient wants to save energy for work and not use it up in the morning trying to get dressed. Allowing the patient to make this choice BEST exemplifies which of the core values and attitudes of occupational therapy?
    a. Altruism
    b. Dignity
    c. Equality
    d. Freedom

39. The contract therapist is working in the schools this week. Where would the therapist look to find the school-based OT's treatment plan for a third grader with severe learning disabilities and hearing impairment?
    a. Individualized Education Plan (IEP)
    b. Individualized Family Service Plan
    c. 504 plan
    d. 700 form

40. An OT is doing a job match search for an injured worker whose functional capacity evaluation recommended "sedentary work" as defined by the *Dictionary of Occupational Titles*. Which job requirements BEST reflect sedentary work?
    a. Exerting up to 5 pounds of force frequently; no walking or standing
    b. Exerting up to 10 pounds of force occasionally; walking and standing occasionally
    c. Exerting up to 15 pounds of force occasionally; 10 pounds of force frequently; 5 pounds of force constantly
    d. Exerting up to 20 pounds of force rarely; standing and walking <50% of the day

41. The most relaxed line of sight with the head erect is 10–15 degrees below the horizontal plane. Using ergonomic principles for

comfortable visual reach, where should the OT recommend that the employee put the list of codes that are frequently needed while typing at the computer?

a. Taped to the monitor above the screen
b. Taped to the desk surface to the left of the keyboard
c. Taped to the monitor below the screen
d. Printed on the mouse pad

42. The owner of Acme Factory consulted an OT for advice on where to place the safety off switch on a new machine. The owner wants it to be as high as possible. The employees are predominantly men and range in height from 5–6 feet tall. What is an appropriate height for the button that will be accessible to all the employees?

a. 60 inches from ground
b. 70 inches from ground
c. 80 inches from ground
d. 90 inches from ground

43. A child who is withdrawn has an occupational therapy goal of increasing ability to express feelings. Which intervention strategy would MOST effectively promote this skill?

a. Drawing a self-portrait
b. Talking about feelings in a small group of peers
c. Playing a video game familiar to the child
d. Watching a movie about a child with similar psychosocial behavior

44. To promote visual tracking for a preschooler who has poor tracking skills, which recommendation is the MOST appropriate for the OT to make to the parents for a home program?

a. Throwing and catching a ball
b. Catching and bursting soap bubbles
c. Playing softball
d. Tossing and catching water balloons

45. A child in middle school has Duchenne's muscular dystrophy. The child uses a manual wheelchair for short distances but is often late and fatigued on arriving to class. The BEST recommendation the OT could make for the use of the wheelchair in school is:

a. Have a peer push the student to all classes
b. Continue to use the manual wheelchair for upper extremity strengthening
c. Explore obtaining an electric wheelchair
d. Ask teachers to forgive the student's lateness to class

46. A 7-year-old with a diagnosis of mild mental retardation is learning to tie their shoes in therapy at school. To reinforce and facilitate generalization of the skill, the OT recommends:
    a. That the parents purchase brightly-colored shoe laces
    b. Fitting the child's shoes with Velcro closures
    c. Having the child practice shoe tying at home
    d. Providing elastic shoe laces

47. A child who has developmental delays has learned to hold the scissors correctly and can snip paper. What is the NEXT scissor activity to upgrade the child's skills?
    a. Cut out squiggly shapes
    b. Cut out large circles and squares
    c. Cut out paper dolls with various shapes
    d. Cut on wide pre-drawn straight lines

48. Goals for children in school should be written in terms of classroom behaviors needed for academic performance. Which is an example of a goal reflecting this thinking?
    a. The student will maintain prone extension posture over a therapy ball in 2 out of 3 trials by the end of the grading period.
    b. When engaged in written assignments in class, the student will maintain an upright sitting posture without verbal cues in 2 of 3 observations.
    c. The student will point to all lowercase *m*s on a candy wrapper within 5 minutes in 2 out of 3 trials.
    d. To increase upper extremity strength, the student will lift 2-pound weights with 10 repetitions bilaterally in 2 out of 3 trials.

49. A community outing of bowling is planned for a group of elderly patients from a day care center. Neuromuscular factors that the OT must consider before engaging in the activity are:
    a. Cognition and ability to follow instructions
    b. Strength, coordination, and endurance
    c. Attention span and hearing ability
    d. Visual scanning and tracking

50. An OT in a community center would like to select the best activity to facilitate socialization and to increase several participants' energy level. The BEST choice would be:
    a. A chair aerobic group
    b. A cooking group
    c. A card game tournament
    d. A walk along a path in the park

51. Through an occupational therapy profile, the OT discovers that an elderly client recently lost a spouse for whom the client was the primary caregiver. Which is the BEST intervention strategy to address the client's use of time?
    a. Suggest visiting with church members and family
    b. Organize the client's friends to go shopping
    c. Provide an opportunity for volunteering
    d. Mention sleeping as a way of avoiding thinking about the loss

52. Occupational therapy potentially may have to address aging issues in these three categories:
    a. Parental, biological, and psychological
    b. Psychological, chronological, and parental
    c. Chronological, biological, and social
    d. Parental, social, and biological

53. An 85-year-old client with normal age-related physical changes will have the MOST cardiovascular stress with which of the following activities?
    a. Brushing teeth at the sink while holding onto the counter
    b. Getting dressed while sitting on the edge of the bed
    c. Walking to the mailbox 250 feet from the house
    d. Carrying a basket of laundry from the basement

54. An elderly client presents with an ulnar nerve injury, for which the OT fabricates a splint. The therapist must take into consideration which of the following goals?
    a. Assist function of the thumb for tip-to-tip prehension
    b. Assist grasp by providing stability of the wrist in extension
    c. Prevent clawing and assist in grasp and release
    d. Prevent overstretching the wrist extensors

55. A 3-year-old child with a diagnosis of developmental coordination disorder is being seen in a private clinic for Sensory Integration–based occupational therapy. The OT sets up an obstacle course with tunnels and cones. The OT encourages the child to explore it. It is MOST likely that the OT is trying to:
    a. Support the child's development of adaptive motor responses in novel situations
    b. Assess whether or not the child demonstrates an aversive response to having both feet off the ground
    c. Provide the child with opportunities to increase trunk and upper extremity strength
    d. Help the child develop essential preacademic skills

56. The OT is providing services in the school system and is asked to provide consultation to a teacher who has a student with a

hearing impairment in the classroom. The teacher knows that the child can lip read and consults with the OT in preparation for the student. After listening to the teacher's concerns, the OT provides some recommendations. One recommendation the OT might make to the teacher is to:

a. Limit the amount of verbal interactions between the teacher and the student
b. Avoid standing in front of the window while conducting a lesson
c. Exaggerate mouth movements when speaking to the student
d. Seat the child in the back of the classroom

57. The OT is working in the hospital with an 8-year-old child who has burns over 70% of the body. During the initial acute phase of treatment, the OT's primary objective is to:

a. Assess the child's community participation skills
b. Return the child to developmentally appropriate levels of play
c. Prevent loss of joint mobility
d. Educate the parent on how to advocate for the child's needs when returning to school

58. The OT is providing service at school to a 4-year-old patient with arthrogryposis. The child's goal is to increase independence with self-feeding. The OT believes that the child will be more successful if using adaptive equipment during lunchtime. It is likely that the OT will recommend that this child use:

a. Built-up utensils
b. A non-slip placemat
c. An augmentative communication device
d. Long handled utensils

59. The OT is providing service to a 10-year-old patient with spina bifida to address toileting at school. The patient is incontinent and has expressed embarrassment to the teacher and the OT. It is likely that the OT will recommend:

a. That the student use the toilet at regular intervals throughout the day
b. That the teacher and student will work out a signal when the student wants to use the bathroom
c. That the child wear pants with an elastic waistband so that they can be pulled down quickly
d. That the child only go to the bathroom when the other students in the class go

60. The OT is working with an 11-year-old child who complains of hand fatigue after writing 2–3 short sentences. After observing the child complete a handwriting task, the OT discovers that the child uses an efficient grip but exerts an increased amount of pressure when writing. To address this issue, the OT might recommend that the child:
    a. Dictate the answers
    b. Use a built-up pencil grip to maintain the use of an efficient grasp
    c. Write on a surface that provides the child with more feedback
    d. Use a keyboard to eliminate writing tasks

61. The OT is working with an 8-year-old patient who has a diagnosis of attention deficit disorder (ADD). At school, the patient often gets in trouble for walking around the room and finds it difficult to sit and work for long periods of time. The OT might recommend that:
    a. The child use color-coded folders to organize the various different subjects.
    b. The teacher discuss with the child's parents the possibility of medication to control the increased energy level.
    c. The child stand at a counter in the back of the room to complete assigned work.
    d. The child use an assignment notebook to record all assignments that were missed while the child was wandering around the classroom.

62. The OT is helping a child who is in the second grade hold a pencil by using just three digits. The OT notices that child lacks stability on the ulnar side of the hand making it difficult to functionally hold the pencil with the first three digits. It is likely that the OT will try to encourage the child to:
    a. Hold a small paper clip against the palmar side of the hand with the fourth and fifth digits while maintaining a three digit pencil grasp
    b. Hold the pencil with a four digit grasp and the use of a built-up pencil gripper
    c. Try writing with the other hand
    d. Participate in craft projects that require tearing paper and spreading paste

63. When treating a child for issues related to feeding, the OT wants more information related to the child's respiratory control. It is likely that the OT will refer the child to a:
    a. Gastrointestinal specialist
    b. Pulmonary specialist
    c. Otolaryngologist
    d. Neurologist

64. The OT is working in early intervention with a 34-month-old child. The OT will be assessing the child as part of the transition from early intervention to the school systems. The OT would like to work one-on-one with the child and assess the child's abilities in the following skill areas: object manipulation, grasping, and visual motor integration. It is likely that the OT will choose:
    a. An assessment that measures eye-hand coordination skills
    b. A global assessment that measures motor skill development
    c. An assessment that measures a child's ability to participate in self-care, mobility, and social functions
    d. An assessment that measures fine and gross motor skills

65. While reviewing a child's past medical history, the OT learns that the child has difficulty with visual pursuit. This child would also need intervention for:
    a. The ability to continue fixation on a moving object to maintain a continuous image
    b. The ability to rapidly change fixation from one point in the visual field to another
    c. The ability to fix eyes on a stationary object
    d. The ability to put forth conscious mental effort to concentrate on a visual task

66. The OT is working with a third-grade student on handwriting. The OT is asking the child to copy a sentence from the chalkboard to the paper. The OT notices that the child writes down one letter at a time and then looks back to the chalkboard to complete one sentence. The child is MOST likely experiencing difficulty with:
    a. Visual closure
    b. Selective attention
    c. Visual memory
    d. Figure-ground

67. A 7-year-old child with sensory integration dysfunction is working with an OT on the school's playground. The child looks at all of the playground equipment and verbalizes a detailed plan on how to move across the various obstacles. When asked to execute these actions, the child had difficulty making the body do what was conceptualized. The OT needs to address sensory integration dysfunction related to:
    a. Somatodyspraxia
    b. Gravitational insecurity
    c. Modulation
    d. Tactile defensiveness

68. The OT evaluated a first-grade student with mild left hemiparesis. Results from the occupational therapy evaluation indicate that

the student is able to independently participate in all aspects of the educational environment, including physical education with few adaptations. At this child's IEP meeting, it is likely that the therapist will:

a. Recommend direct service to address concerns regarding the child's ability to independently bathe at home

b. Not recommend any service because other members of the team can recommend additional adaptations and modifications

c. Recommend direct service to address the child's tone and the development of age-appropriate hand skills

d. Not recommend direct service because the child is independent at school

69. The OT is working with a 9-year-old student in the school system. The child has adequate upper extremity control but limited fine motor control and dexterity making handwriting difficult. The OT would like to introduce keyboarding to the student but knows that a standard keyboard will not support success with the task. It is likely that the OT will choose:

a. A head mouse

b. A mini-keyboard

c. An expanded keyboard

d. A voice activated software program

70. A medically fragile infant is being discharged from the hospital and evaluated for home-based early intervention services. The family requests that after all team members assess the child, only one or two professionals actually come in to the house to provide service to their infant. This approach to service provision can BEST be described as:

a. Intradisciplinary

b. Community based

c. Interdisciplinary

d. Transdisciplinary

71. A child has difficulty holding a fork during self-feeding because of decreased sensory receptors in the hand. The OT will MOST likely recommend the use of:

a. A weighted utensil

b. A utensil with a cuff

c. A larger utensil

d. A textured utensil

72. A school-aged child with figure-ground concerns is being seen in occupational therapy. The OT will MOST likely recommend that the classroom teacher:

a. Place a red line on the left side of the paper
b. Use a frame to block out all areas of the page except for the information that the child is supposed to be focusing on
c. Provide the child with a copy of all notes that are written on the chalkboard
d. Allow the student to use a highlighter marker

73. An OT is working with a young child who has a diagnosis of a TBI and presents with poor postural alignment and increased tone unilaterally. The OT is working in the neurodevelopmental treatment frame of reference and is concerned because the child presents with decreased degrees of freedom at the shoulder joint. In this situation, prolonged fixing can MOST likely lead to:
a. Impaired sensation in the affected extremity
b. Decreased ROM at joints distal to the shoulder
c. Contracture at the shoulder joint
d. Dissociation of movement patterns

74. A 7-year-old child with an autism spectrum disorder has difficulty making eye contact. The BEST way for the OT working with the child to encourage the child to make eye contact is to:
a. Provide positive reinforcement when the child does engage in eye contact
b. Manually turn the child's head so that the child must look at the OT
c. Give a verbal direction paired with a visual support
d. Ask a peer to model the desired behavior or response

75. An OT is training a caregiver to position an 18-month-old child with low tone in a sidelyer so that the child can explore a toy. Provided that the child does not have scoliosis, the OT will MOST likely recommend that the caregiver position the child:
a. So that the weaker side is on the upside and more mobile
b. For equal amounts of time on both sides throughout the day
c. So that the child's weaker arm is on the downside
d. So that the downside leg is flexed at the knee and the upside leg is extended

76. A school-based OT is working on handwriting with a student who has difficulty maintaining sustained attention. The BEST approach that the OT can use to increase the student's vigilance in therapy is to provide the student with:

    a. Novel materials and numerous activities that encourage the generalization of learned skills

    b. An opportunity to engage in a task that will take the entire session

    c. Repetitive materials that the student is accustomed to and encourage the student to attend to the familiar

    d. Activities that are process driven and do not require goal-oriented attention

77. An OT working in early intervention is helping a parent to get the baby to hold and drink from a bottle. Based on typical development, the therapist should begin to introduce this skill between:
    a. 12–14 months
    b. 10–12 months
    c. 8–10 months
    d. 6–8 months

78. A school-based OT is working with a third-grade student who has difficulty with handwriting. Before working on handwriting at a table in the back of the classroom, the OT should FIRST be sure that the child is positioned:
    a. So that the table is at the child's wrist height
    b. So that the table is at the child's elbow height
    c. So that the table is at the child's shoulder height
    d. In a slightly reclined position at the desk

79. When developing a home program for a child with decreased hand and arm strength, the OT will MOST likely suggest that the child is presented with opportunities to:
    a. Sort dried beans
    b. Play board games
    c. Finger paint
    d. Stir cookie dough

80. After 3 months of intervention, the OT notices that the child is beginning to integrate the reflex that turns the head toward the child's extended arm while in prone. This reflex is:
    a. Asymmetric tonic neck reflex
    b. Symmetric tonic neck reflex
    c. Moro reflex
    d. Tonic labyrinthine reflex

81. A young child is working in occupational therapy on increasing visual–motor integration skills by tracing on a line with a marker. To further address this goal, the OT may also encourage the child to:
     a. Hop up and down
     b. Build a cube tower
     c. Match a picture to an object
     d. Imitate motor movements without verbal cues

82. A child is hospitalized related to complications from cystic fibrosis (CF). Inpatient occupational therapy will MOST likely focus on teaching the child:
     a. Active ROM
     b. Strengthening activities
     c. Energy conservation techniques
     d. Ways to compensate for decreased balance

83. A child with spina bifida uses a variety of different positioning devices throughout the day. The OT would like the child to be in a stander during their treatment session. The OT will MOST likely choose to position the child in:
     a. A mobile stander
     b. A prone stander
     c. A supine stander
     d. A hydraulic stander

84. The OT is working in the school systems with the 18- to 21-year-old population. The focus of occupational therapy is MOST likely to address:
     a. Educational goals
     b. Transition goals
     c. Leisure goals
     d. Self-care goals

85. The OT is leading a group of children in an early childhood classroom. The OT is working with the children on their cutting skills. Before being able to cut a piece of paper in half, the children must be able to:
     a. Trace their names
     b. Cut on thin lines
     c. Snip with scissors
     d. Tear cardboard

86. The OT is working with a left-handed child on letter formation. The OT should cue the child to slant the writing paper so that it is parallel to:
     a. The right forearm when the child is securing the writing paper with the nondominant hand
     b. The top of the desk

   c.   The left forearm when the child's forearm is resting on the desk and in a neutral position

   d.   The left forearm when the child's forearms are both resting on the desk and the child's hands are clasped

87.   The OT is educating a caregiver on how to carry a 30-pound child with severe spasticity who is in a predominantly flexed position. It is MOST likely that the OT will recommend that:

   a.   The caregiver position the child so that both of the child's legs wrap around the caregiver's waist; the caregiver should support the child with one hand under one buttock and the other hand high on the child's back.

   b.   The caregiver position the child so that the child is on its side with its back up against the caregiver's stomach; coming from behind, the caregiver should hold the child by positioning one arm between the child's legs with one hand supporting the child at its stomach and the other arm wrapping around the child's chest and the other hand supporting the child at the elbow.

   c.   The caregiver position the child over the caregiver's shoulder with the child's arms tucked down at its sides and its legs fully extended.

   d.   The child be carried like a cradled baby with the caregiver supporting the child with both hands under its buttocks.

88.   You are observing another therapist in your clinic area instructing a patient who has sustained a brain injury in using association. You know the therapist is using a remediation technique to address a deficit in:

   a.   Attention

   b.   Memory

   c.   Scanning

   d.   Motor planning

89.   You are working with a 60-year-old patient who has sustained a cerebrovascular accident (CVA). The patient presents with low muscle tone. You are working on neuromuscular re-education and utilizing a Rood approach by helping the patient position himself on hands and knees and asking the patient to do an activity with the stronger arm. By doing this you are utilizing:

   a.   Proprioceptive facilitatory techniques of joint compression

   b.   Proprioceptive facilitatory technique of vestibular stimulation

   c.   Inhibitory technique of joint compression

   d.   Inhibitory technique of neutral warmth

90.   According to Bobath, the BEST way to regulate increased flexor tone of the upper extremity is by:

   a.   Positioning the pelvis forward

   b.   Positioning the body in supine

   c.   Weight bearing over the involved upper extremity

   d.   Trunk rotation

91. When instructing a hemiplegic patient on dressing techniques, it is very important that the patient is instructed in which of the following?
    a. The weaker arm or leg is dressed first
    b. The stronger arm or leg is dressed first
    c. Clothes with elastic are easier to wear
    d. Clothes a size larger than usual are easier to wear

92. According to Bobath, the MOST effective way to encourage movement when treating a subluxed shoulder is to use a:
    a. Sling
    b. Taping
    c. Proper positioning
    d. All of the above

93. When facilitating movement in a patient who has sustained a CVA, you use the technique of tapping the wrist extensors. This would come from:
    a. Brunnstrom
    b. Bobath
    c. Proprioceptive neuromuscular facilitation
    d. None of the above

94. A patient who suffered a minor stroke is referred to outpatient occupational therapy with approval for only two visits. Based on the set time limit to see this patient, the focus of treatment will be determined based on the client's:
    a. Most significant client factor deficit
    b. Level of independence in occupational performance areas
    c. Stated goals
    d. History and needs of the family

95. The OT evaluated a patient in the cardiac intensive care unit and is in the process of developing the intervention plan. What are the two primary components that should be included?
    a. The anticipated outcome and the methods to achieve those outcomes
    b. Rehab potential and realistic time frame for seeing the patient
    c. Specific intervention techniques and rationale for being chosen
    d. The type of tests given and interpretation of the results

96. A patient with fibromyalgia has performance deficits in ADLs, including lack of a daily routine because of a loss of energy and motivation to engage in daily occupations, depression and anxiety, and difficulty managing home and instrumental activities of daily living (IADL) because of fatigue and pain. Based on these performance deficits, the initial focus of treatment should be:

   a. Completing IADL tasks independently

   b. Establishing a new daily routine that can be done within the patient's tolerance

   c. Referring to a support group to address depression and anxiety

   d. Energy conservation and activities for pain management

97. The goal of treatment for a patient with impaired sensation is to promote touch localization to improve interpretation of tactile sensation with work activities. During a sensory re-education program, the OT should emphasize:

   a. Activities related to stereognosis

   b. Distinguishing hot and cold temperatures

   c. Graphesthesia and identifying moving and static stimuli

   d. Topographic orientation

98. The BEST example of a statement that would be documented in the assessment portion of a subjective, objective, assessment, and plan (SOAP) note is:

   a. Client and spouse participated in a discussion about planning activities of interest for the patient.

   b. Client complains of difficulty donning night-time splint and requests that the splint be re-evaluated by the therapist.

   c. Family was referred to social services for consideration of alternative placement.

   d. Client demonstrates good understanding of the home program but requires supervision to perform independently.

99. Which is the BEST means for documenting a goal statement?

   a. Therapist will instruct the patient in overhead dressing techniques.

   b. Patient will participate in meal preparation for 15 minutes without breaks.

   c. Patient will perform 10 repetitions of active assistive shoulder ladder exercises.

   d. Patient will show increased endurance for performing ADLs.

100. Which statement would be the MOST appropriate for the OT to document in the plan section of the SOAP note?

   a. Client given educational materials to practice correcting posture and trunk balance during daily routine.

   b. Client able to respond to verbal instructions and questions with correct responses 3 out of 3 times.

   c. Client indicates that the long-term goal is to return to work on a full time basis.

   d. Client assessed for use of in compensatory techniques while cooking in the clinic kitchen.

101. An office worker has thoracic outlet syndrome. What modifications might the occupational therapy consultant recommend for the workstation?
  a. Place any overhead items near the front of the shelf to minimize full extension when reaching
  b. When sitting at the desk, use a chair with arm rests to allow support to the upper extremities
  c. Place heavier items furthest away on the desk surface
  d. Place lighter items furthest away on the desk surface

102. A patient recently underwent a rotator cuff repair. The BEST instruction to provide to a patient whose goal is to be independent in dressing as soon a possible is to:
  a. Use one-handed technique for dressing
  b. Proceed with use of both cautiously while dressing
  c. Proceed as normal as there are no restrictions
  d. Use the affected extremity as an active assist

103. A teenager with a history of juvenile rheumatoid arthritis (JRA) needs to manage the medications routine. The teenager inquires about typical side effects of the medications. The OT should refer the teenager to information related to:
  a. Antidepressants
  b. Nonsteroidal anti-inflammatory drugs
  c. Anticoagulants
  d. Barbiturates

104. A patient with a total shoulder arthroplasty has been receiving therapy for 1 week. The patient has achieved pain-free ROM to within functional limits. The OT should progress treatment to include:
  a. Lifting activities
  b. Initiation of activities in standing
  c. IADL
  d. Activities involving speed, such as throwing a ball

105. The OT should instruct a patient with de Quervain's tenosynovitis to minimize functional activities involving:
  a. Reaching overhead
  b. Grasping
  c. Forced pinch
  d. Total arm extension

106. An OT is working to facilitate motor skills and control with a group of patients that have Parkinson's disease. The BEST activity to use is:

     a. Bowling
     b. Card game tournament
     c. Gardening
     d. Rhythmic musical game

107. A stand pivot transfer would be used for a client when the client:
     a. Can come to standing and weight shift while the therapist secures the client with a transfer belt
     b. Is learning to use a walker for ambulation
     c. Is able to do some, but not full, weight bearing on one or both legs
     d. Has lower extremities that are too weak for weight bearing

108. In providing instructions and training to a family for a person that will require assistance in transfers, the OT should tell them that when performing transfers:
     a. Allow the client to put the arms around the neck of the person performing the transfer and pull to stand
     b. Stand behind the patient and push the individual forward
     c. Keep the back and spine straight as possible and lift or rotate using the arm muscles
     d. Keep the back curved so as not to put pressure on the legs when lifting

109. A patient with fibromyalgia lives alone and is a meticulous housekeeper; however, the patient cannot hire anyone to assist with household chores because of financial resources. During a home visit, the patient requests advice on the best method to perform household duties. The OT should recommend that the patient:
     a. Schedule homemaking chores so that heavy tasks are alternated during the week
     b. Invite friends and neighbors to assist with some of the heavier tasks on an alternating basis
     c. Seek funding from social services to hire in-home assistance for household chores
     d. Consider attending a support group to deal with the limitations of this condition

110. For a patient with cognitive deficits, intervention is organized around four phases. The MOST advanced phase of cognitive retraining should involve:
     a. Anticipation
     b. Application
     c. Adaptation
     d. Acquisition

111. The OT in a skilled nursing facility is asked to recommend the best type of clothing to facilitate dressing for the general patient population. The OT would MOST likely recommend:
    a. Loose fitting garments that can be pulled overhead
    b. Garments that have a combination of elastic and buttons or zipper closures
    c. Front opening, firm fitting garment without excess fabric and zipper closures
    d. Front opening, loose fitting garments with large fasteners or Velcro closures

112. Intervention planning involves writing goals to guide the intervention process. Select the MOST appropriate written goal for a client who can no longer do laundry because of lower back pain:
    a. The patient will be instructed in techniques to do tasks related to laundry without pain.
    b. The patient will use work simplification techniques and proper body mechanics to do laundry independently.
    c. The patient will be taught work simplification tasks to be able to do laundry.
    d. The patient will be independent when performing laundry tasks.

113. An occupational therapy consultant is asked to recommend equipment using universal design principles to incorporate in a retirement village. What approach might the OT take?
    a. Assess the potential residents and recommend customized equipment based on each person's needs
    b. Recommend installing special lifts in the housing units with stairs
    c. Recommend items that eliminate barriers, such as widening doors or lowering counters
    d. Suggest installing voice control for lights and doors

114. The OT is working with a patient to increase arousal and attentiveness. The patient has mastered the ability to visually attend. The OT should NEXT incorporate:
    a. Identifying objects
    b. Imitation of postures
    c. Figure-ground activities
    d. Visual tracking

115. After the evaluation, the OT recommends that the patient work on dressing skills and basic ADLs. However, the patient indicates that these are tasks that the spouse can assist with; the patient would rather concentrate on re-establishing leisure pursuits. What action should be taken by the OT?

    a. Insist the patient perform basic ADLs as this will be helpful to the spouse

    b. Bargain with the patient to work on both areas

    c. Switch emphasis of treatment based on client's preferences

    d. Refuse treatment because the patient and therapist disagree

116. In inpatient cardiac rehab, the OT should concentrate on:

    a. Educating about risk factors and appropriate home activities for discharge

    b. Maximizing psychosocial and vocational status in the community

    c. Assessing the ability to resume occupation related to job performance

    d. Establishing a daily exercise routine to build strength and endurance

117. The goal of therapy for a patient is to develop and improve hand coordination and skills. The OT should recommend purposeful activities, such as:

    a. Games, crafts, and self-care tasks

    b. Using Thera-Putty and hand gripper

    c. Cone stacking and placing pegs in a board

    d. Playing a "clapping game"

118. To bill Medicare Part B for a piece of adapted equipment, such as a wheelchair, the OT must document that the:

    a. Equipment will enable independent functioning

    b. Patient has secondary insurance for co-pay

    c. Equipment is medically necessary

    d. Equipment was ordered by the physician

119. The OT should avoid isometric strengthening as a prelude to functional activities for patients with:

    a. Diabetes

    b. Cumulative trauma disorders

    c. Cardiovascular problems

    d. Arthritis

120. An OT is writing a functional problem list. Which of the following should be included?

    a. Decreased ROM of the upper extremities

    b. Deceased muscle strength at a grade of fair minus

    c. Swelling of right upper extremity

    d. Limited ability to grasp because of edema

121. A client with scleroderma is being seen for a home program. Using the Model of Human Occupation as a frame of

reference, the OT evaluation of the individual should focus primarily on:
a. The problem areas and deficits
b. Clarification of thoughts, feelings, and experiences that influence behavior
c. Cognitive function, including assets and limitations
d. The impact of personal traits and the environment on role performance

122. During a family conference, the OT recommends a large piece of adapted equipment that the patient will need when discharged. The family would like to obtain the equipment but is concerned about the expense. In advising the family, the OT should use this type of reasoning:
a. Narrative
b. Scientific
c. Ethical
d. Pragmatic

123. Because of frequent bouts of weakness, an individual requires help approximately 60% to 70% of the time getting into and out of bed and going to the bathroom. When instructing the caregiver on the level of help the person will need, the OT would recommend:
a. Minimum assistance
b. Moderate assistance
c. Maximum assistance
d. Constant supervision

124. A patient with a head injury is confused at times but demonstrates appropriate behaviors and is responsive to others. The individual is also scheduled for discharge, and the family will need a home program for basic ADLs and safety. The OT should advise the family to:
a. Perform self-care tasks for the individual and provide constant supervision for safety
b. Provide assistance with self-care tasks and frequently supervise for safety
c. Provide cueing and directions for self-care tasks and minimal supervision for safety
d. Encourage the individual to perform self-care when confusion is at a minimum to ensure safety

125. A patient with a head injury demonstrates confusion and constant agitation. The occupational therapy intervention should focus on:
a. Self-care skills
b. Attention span and safety
c. Sequencing and organizing tasks
d. Functional transfers

126. A patient with a diagnosis of a TBI exhibits inappropriate episodic outbursts and has difficulty with concentration, memory, and following directions for ADLs and IADLs. What frame of reference would guide the OT in determining the BEST treatment approach?
    a. Rehabilitation
    b. Biomechanical
    c. Neurodevelopmental
    d. Cognitive behavioral

127. A 55-year-old patient with osteoporosis is being discharged from acute care with functional independence in all occupational performance areas. What discharge recommendations would be appropriate for this individual?
    a. Provide a list of alternatives for leisure pursuits
    b. Recommend that a family member take over driving responsibilities
    c. Instruct on in-home safety and energy conservation
    d. Provide alternative instructions on how to perform self-care

128. An individual with a TBI has difficulty with auditory processing. When communicating with the individual, the OT should:
    a. Move to quiet environment
    b. Speak slowly
    c. Use visual cures
    d. Have person use a hearing aid

129. An adolescent has been admitted to your unit with a diagnosis of conduct disorder. Substance abuse is also suspected. The client is capable of meeting all the basic needs but maladaptive behavior is disrupting performance. The MOST appropriate occupational therapy goal for a treatment plan would be that the patient will:
    a. Become independent in ADLs by end of week by taking a shower without assistance every day for 5 consecutive days
    b. Attend OT group for 2 weeks and choose a vocational pursuit by the end of week two and develop a plan for the necessary schooling, etc
    c. Demonstrate appropriate group behavior, such as waiting the patient's turn, raising a hand to speak, etc., in all occupational therapy groups for 1 week
    d. Not curse

130. You have received an order for ADL training for a newly admitted adolescent with conduct disorder. The written order came from a new medicine resident that is unfamiliar with psychiatric occupational therapy services. From your first observation it is

obvious that this adolescent has no need for ADL training. Your NEXT step would be to:
a. Go ahead and follow the order as written
b. Ignore the order and do what is more appropriate for the patient as a qualified professional
c. Confront and tell the doctor that you are going to educate the doctor
d. Ask to speak with the doctor, briefly explain occupational therapy services, and discuss rewriting the order so that you can evaluate the patient's occupational therapy needs and treat accordingly

131. Your patient is refusing all groups. You would:
a. Realize that you can't make the patient go and remove the patient from your caseload
b. Tell the patient that it's mandatory and the doctor said that the patient has to participate
c. Get the nurse to make the patient go
d. Ask the patient to tell you why they do not want to participate

132. A preadolescent presents with social immaturity and problems socializing. Which of the following goals would BEST meet the client's needs?
a. Patient will initiate and engage independently in a 15-minute structured game, with one peer, by the end of the third occupational therapy session.
b. Patient will initiate making the bed each day for five consecutive days.
c. Patient will talk at length about the parent–patient relationship and feelings about having no childhood friends.
d. Patient will share all feelings with the group.

133. In evaluating a new geriatric patient, you note that the patient spends most of the day in front of the television. The patient tells you that the TV watching has been going on ever since the patient's spouse died 5 years ago. An appropriate goal to set might be:
a. Patient will explore possible leisure options in occupational therapy sessions, to help improve life balance and increase socialization and will pick 2 new activities to begin participating in by the end of the week.
b. Patient will watch only 2 hours of television each day.
c. Patient will stop sitting around and start doing things.
d. Patient will talk about the loss of the spouse in occupational therapy groups.

134. Which of the following is the BEST example of a functional goal in school-based occupational therapy?

  a. The student will stack eight 1-inch blocks, 4 of 5 trials, by the end of the semester.

  b. The student will place 5 pegs in a pegboard, 2 of 3 trials, by the end of the semester.

  c. The student will use a visual schedule to independently transition between class activities, 80% of the time, by end of the semester.

  d. The student will cut along a line with scissors by the end of the semester.

135. Which of the following skills is considered the BEST predictor of handwriting ability?
  a. Letter recognition
  b. Visual perceptual
  c. Hand dominance
  d. Visual–motor

136. At what age should children be expected to begin to cut a simple circle or square with scissors?
  a. 1–2 years
  b. 2–3 years
  c. 3–5 years
  d. 5–6 years

137. Important considerations for the IEP team in determining the need for occupational therapy as a related service would include each of the following except:
  a. The results and recommendations of an occupational therapy evaluation
  b. Whether the problem requires the unique expertise of an OT
  c. Whether the problem interferes with the student's participation in the educational program
  d. Whether the student's classroom has an aide to follow through on OT suggestions

138. Which of the following is the MOST significant factor in determining if a student should receive school-based occupational therapy services?
  a. IEP team decision
  b. Occupational therapy evaluation results
  c. Insurance coverage
  d. Parent preference

139. Which of the following is the MOST appropriate example of a task an OT may delegate to classroom staff for a student with identified sensory integration differences?

a. Physically applying a vibrating toy to a student
b. Requiring a student to go down the slide a set number of times while on the playground
c. Monitoring a student in completing a written sensory diet of heavy work activities
d. Spinning a student on a swing

140. Which of the following could a school-based OT use that would MOST appropriately allow parents to routinely express concerns to the OT?
a. Individualized handouts including pictures or diagrams
b. A home program designed to fit into the family's routine
c. Attendance at the annual IEP team meeting
d. Notebook sent back and forth between a school-based OT and parents

141. Which of the following would be an appropriate goal for a school-based OT applying the sensory integration framework?
a. The student will swing on therapy swing for 60 seconds without signs of distress by end of the 6 weeks.
b. The student will demonstrate decreased signs of tactile defensiveness by end of semester.
c. The student will improve body awareness by wearing a weighted vest as prescribed by therapist, daily.
d. The student will independently choose a coping strategy to use when cued by the classroom staff by end of 6 weeks.

142. What is the primary resource a school-based OT uses in determining the frames of reference and interventions MOST appropriate to meet team identified educationally relevant goals?
a. Outpatient therapy goals
b. Occupational therapy assistant observations
c. Clinical reasoning
d. Teaching style used in the classroom

143. A parent reports that their child sleeps pushed up against the sides of the crib. The parent states that the child pushes hard into one end of the crib. The OT realizes that this child requires treatment that focuses on:
a. Proprioceptive input of deep pressure
b. Vestibular input of spinning
c. Light touch
d. Kinesthetic input

144. A patient with rheumatoid arthritis has been receiving therapy for 2 weeks to work on strengthening and fine motor skills to improve occupational performance in the areas of cooking, manipulation of fasteners for dressing, and the performance of leisure tasks, such as playing cards and board games. Today, the patient arrives in an exacerbated state with swollen inflamed joints. The OT should:

    a. Modify treatment to focus on performing light leisure activities such as playing cards and board games
    b. Continue current treatment but reduce the time frame of the treatment session
    c. Discontinue treatment and reschedule when inflammation has subsided
    d. Modify treatment to focus on resting of joints and engage in light activities as tolerated

Answers to Intervention Planning Questions

1. d. Occupational therapists (OTs) should listen with empathy to understand family concerns and needs, explain the constraints of the system when the parents' requests cannot be met, make adaptations to services based on the parents' input, and suggest alternative resources to parents when their requests cannot be met within the system. The OT should also verbally acknowledge family priorities and discuss parents' suggestions and requests with administrators to increase the possibilities that policies and agency structure can change to benefit families. The parents should be provided with the information about their child in a supportive manner. *Occupational Therapy for Children* by Case-Smith

2. a. A tenodesis splint uses active wrist extension to aid in passive finger flexion or grasp. When the wrist is flexed, this facilitates the opposite action or finger release. This is a common technique for promoting grasp and release for persons with C6–7 spinal cord injuries. *Introduction to Splinting: A Clinical Reasoning and Problem Solving Approach* by Coppard and Lohman

3. c. The functional hand position, also called the midpoint position, is used to promote rest of the hand, functional alignment, and functional hand patterns, such as opposition and grasp. Although some positions may vary slightly, the placement for the functional hand position is wrist in 20–30 degrees, thumb in 45 degrees palmar abduction, metacarpophalengeals in 35–45 degrees of flexion, and the interphalengeals in slight flexion. *Introduction to Splinting: A Clinical Reasoning and Problem Solving Approach* by Coppard and Lohman

4. c. Fractured sites should remain stable to promote healing and realignment of the bones. However, the OT should encourage the movement of adjacent joints to assist in maintaining muscle strength and lengthening of tendons and muscles. *Occupational Therapy for Physical Dysfunction* by Trombly and Radomski

5. c. An assisted living facility provides a range of care and services. These facilities are designed to help clients maintain their functional status and provide medical intervention or assistance when needed. *Occupational Therapy in Community-Based Practice* by Scaffa

6. c. According to the definitions on levels of assistance, supervision means standby assistance of one person so that the patient

performs the adapted or therapeutic activity in a safe and effective manner. *Occupational Therapy for Physical Dysfunction* by Trombly and Radomski

7. c. In conditional reasoning, the OT tries to understand what is meaningful to the patient and the patient's perception of both the self and others in a variety of contexts. To be client-centered, contextual factors including culture, social, physical, and spiritual, and their influence must be understood during the assessment. This guides decisions about the intervention. *Occupational Therapy for Physical Dysfunction* by Trombly and Radomski

8. a. The OT should work to control pain before using the involved extremity for functional activities, such as grooming and basic ADLs. Although gentle mobilization may be used, pain management techniques should the immediate focus. Pain management spans a wide array of techniques, including relaxation, massage, biofeedback, and positioning. *Hand Rehabilitation: A Quick Reference Guide and Review* by Weiss and Falkenstein

9. a. Angina is recurring chest pain and is an indication of coronary artery disease. An onset of angina during treatment should be considered an emergency, because of the possibility of a heart attack, and will need to be addressed by the physician. *Occupational Therapy for Physical Dysfunction* by Trombly and Radomski

10. d. Distracters (a), (b), and (c) may be appropriate interventions; however, Alzheimer's disease is progressive in nature. Therefore, with the expected decline and being in the home environment, the OT should focus on educating the primary caregiver on understanding the progressive nature of the disease and strategies for assisting the patient to remain functional as long as possible. *Functional Performance in Older Adults* by Bonder and Wagner

11. b. The social context refers to the organized patterns of behavior that are expected from persons and that pertain to the social interaction with others. *Applying the Occupational Therapy Practice Framework* by Skubik-Peplaski, Paris, Boyle, and Culpert

12. a. The first priority is to reduce edema, because other symptoms may be somewhat relieved and motion can be enhanced with

a reduction in swelling. *Occupational Therapy for Physical Dysfunction* by Trombly and Radomski

13. b. Patients with a TBI may demonstrate impulsive and socially inappropriate behavior. The OT must be alert to these issues, because patients with TBIs often need to undergo a work readiness program focused on retraining in socially appropriate behavior and responses. *Conditions in Occupational Therapy: Effects on Occupational Performance* by Hansen and Atchinson

14. b. The inability to extend the wrist and supinate the forearm affects grasp. This can also be seen with tenodesis action. Wrist extension facilitates finger closure and wrist flexion facilitates opening of the fingers and the hand. This type of issue is typically seen with radial nerve compression or injury. *Introduction to Splinting: A Clinical Reasoning and Problem Solving Approach* by Coppard and Lohman

15. c. If there are no other complications, a person with a spinal cord injury at the level of C8 would most likely be independent in mobility with the use of either a manual or motorized wheelchair and a sliding board for transfers. *Basic Rehabilitation Techniques: A Self Instructional Guide* by Sine, Liss, Roush, Holcomb, and Wilson

16. a. Following hip precautions, it is essential to avoid hyperextension or flexion of the hip past 90 degrees. In a wheelchair, a cushion or pillow should be placed in the seat to reduce the angle of the hip while seated, and the legs should be positioned in neutral to prevent internal or external rotation with the use of an abductor pillow. *Basic Rehabilitation Techniques: A Self Instructional Guide* by Sine, Liss, Roush, Holcomb, and Wilson

17. b. In short-term treatment, the expectation is often not to alter the source of chronic pain but to improve the patient's means of coping with and adapting to pain while improving participation and quality of life. *Basic Rehabilitation Techniques: A Self Instructional Guide* by Sine, Liss, Roush, Holcomb, and Wilson

18. a. The general goal of a pain management program is to return the patient to society at the maximal functional level and with the ability to cope with any residual discomfort in an appropriate manner. *Basic Rehabilitation Techniques: A Self Instructional Guide* by Sine, Liss, Roush, Holcomb, and Wilson

19. d. Increased symptoms related to carpal tunnel syndrome may indicate a need to rest the extremity in a splint to align structures and reduce inflammation and pressure on the structures, such as the median nerve within the carpal tunnel. This will facilitate healing from repetitive use. Therapy should not be discontinued, although the OT should assess and adjust intensity of therapy as needed. *Occupational Therapy Practice Skills for Physical Dysfunction* by Pedretti and Early

20. d. Placing a small weight on the wrist enhances the proprioceptive input when the child moves the arm to engage in functional activities. Therefore, a strategy of augmented and individualized sensory cueing and feedback helps to improve performance. *Occupational Therapy for Children* by Case-Smith

21. a. Cultural values are important to consider when working with children and their families. The OT should attempt to discern the family's view of disability, ideas about discipline, and values for independence versus intradependence. All of these can influence how the family accepts intervention services, what types of intervention strategies should be recommended, how to approach behavioral issues, and how to approach levels and types of service. *Occupational Therapy for Children* by Case-Smith

22. c. Habits, roles, and routines are performance patterns that are adopted by a person as they engage in daily occupation. Habits are often established behavior that provides structure to daily life. *Applying the Occupational Therapy Practice Framework* by Skubik-Peplaski, Paris, Boyle, and Culpert

23. a. Reasonable accommodations are central to the Americans with Disabilities Act (ADA). Reasonable accommodations may include rest breaks, ergonomic interventions, and job modifications. The ADA advocated for persons with disabilities so that attention is paid to access to the workplace for successfully performance of the job. This includes access to the building, workstation, and bathrooms. *Occupational Therapy in Community-Based Practice Settings* by Scaffa

24. c. At the age of 2 years, the child engages in functional or relational play. This means that the child begins to understand the function of an object and that function determines the action. Initially, children use objects on themselves (e.g., pretending to drink from a cup or to comb the hair). These self-directed actions signal the beginning of pretend play. *Occupational Therapy for Children* by Case-Smith

25. c. By the age of 7–8 years, structured games and organized play predominate the play occupations of children. Games with rules are the primary mode for physical and social play. Groups of children organize themselves, assign roles, and explain (or create) rules to guide the game they plan to play. *Occupational Therapy for Children* by Case-Smith

26. d. A child with learning disabilities would usually have primarily cognitive processing issues. Specific learning disabilities include auditory processing, language disabilities, and perceptual disorders. *Occupational Therapy for Children* by Case-Smith

27. b. In home health, the termination of occupational therapy services occurs for three reasons: (1) the goals have been met, (2) the client cannot meet goals based on the OT's judgment, and (3) the person is no longer home bound (i.e., such as meeting friends at a restaurant). *Occupational Therapy in Community-Based Practice Setting* by Scaffa

28. d. Any change in treatment requires notification, discussion with, and approval from a physician. *Occupational Therapy Practice Skills for Physical Dysfunction* by Pedretti and Early

29. a. A mobile arm support is a mechanical device that can stand alone or be attached to a wheelchair. It supports the weight of the shoulders and elbows and allows purposeful movement of these parts of the body to take place. *Occupational Therapy for Physical Dysfunction* by Trombly and Radomski

30. d. MET refers to the amount of energy consumed at rest that is equal to the approximately equivalent to 3.5 milliliters of oxygen per kilogram of body weight per minute. Various tasks or activities require a certain amount of energy to perform. After performing homemaking activities, such as washing dishes and ironing, the next progression in homemaking tasks from the choices listed would be preparing a meal (MET level 3–4). Driving and dressing qualify as a MET level of 2–3; gardening has an MET level of 4–5. *Quick Reference to Occupational Therapy* by Reed

31. c. Splinting and other positioning devices are used to prevent deformity. The three phases of burn healing are emergent (which extends from the initial burn up to 72 hours and focuses on fluid resuscitation), acute (which lasts 72 hours, until the wound closes), and the rehabilitation phase, which begins after

the wound closes and focuses on healing and scar management. *Conditions in Occupational Therapy: Effect on Occupational Performance* by Hansen and Atchinson

32. c. All are viable goals for the OT to address with the patient. However, relief of pain, stiffness, and reduction in inflammation will have a bearing on patient tolerance for other interventions and should be addressed initially. *Conditions in Occupational Therapy: Effect on Occupational Performance* by Hansen and Atchinson

33. d. If grading shoulder flexion, the next step after achieving full shoulder flexion in side lying is to begin to work or perform activities against gravity to begin increasing strength. Shoulder flexion against gravity is achieved with the individual in the sitting or standing position. *Occupational Therapy for Physical Dysfunction* by Trombly and Radomski

34. c. With a problem of hypersensitivity, desensitization is indicated; a partial loss of sensation might mean that sensory retraining is needed. If sensation gets progressively worse and is not expected to return, then compensatory techniques related to safety must be addressed. *Occupational Therapy for Physical Dysfunction* by Trombly and Radomski

35. b. After fabricating and fitting a splint, the OT should have the patient remove the splint after 20–30 minutes of wear and note any pressure marks, redness, or blanching of the skin. Some redness may be common with splint usage; however, it should resolve within 10–15 minutes after removal of the splint. *Occupational Therapy for Physical Dysfunction* by Trombly and Radomski

36. a. This individual would not have the musculature control to complete any of the activities listed but could give verbal directions to an attendant. *Occupational Therapy Practice Skills for Physical Dysfunction* by Pedretti and Early

37. c. The other answers are inconsistent with the Model of Human Occupation and actually apply to other models, that is, the Biomechanical and Motor Control model. *Occupational Therapy Practice Skills for Physical Dysfunction* by Pedretti and Early

38. d. Freedom allows the individual to exercise choice and pursue goals that have personal and social meaning. *Effective Documentation for Occupational Therapy* by AOTA; *Willard & Spackman's Occupational Therapy,* 10th ed. by Crepeau, Cohn, and Schell

39. a. The IEP documents the plan for the student. It is used for students receiving services under the Individuals with Education Act (IDEA). The individualized family service plan is used for children/families receiving early intervention services. A 504 plan is used to help children who do not qualify for services under the IDEA. A 700 form is used in SNFs for Medicare documentation. *Willard & Spackman's Occupational Therapy,* 10th ed. by Crepeau, Cohn, and Schell

40. b. The Dictionary of Occupational Titles defines sedentary work as exerting up to 10 pounds of force occasionally and/or a negligible amount of force frequently or constantly to lift, carry, push, or pull, or otherwise move objects, including the human body. Sedentary work involves sitting most of the time but may involve walking or standing for brief periods of time. *Ergonomics for Therapists* by Jacobs

41. a. The eyes can comfortably rotate about 15 degrees above and below the angle of the relaxed line of sight. Controls or objects needing frequent reading should be placed between 30 degrees below and 5 degrees above the horizontal plane. *Ergonomics for Therapists* by Jacobs

42. b. Maximum arm reach is approximately 2 feet above shoulder height. The highest any button should be is 71 inches if a person is able to stand directly in front of the control panel. *Ergonomics for Therapists* by Jacobs

43. c. Drawing is a task generally understood by children of all ages and can be carried out independently; drawing is a therapeutic technique which provides a child a way to express feelings without the pressures of a group. *Psychosocial Occupational Therapy* by Cara and MacRae

44. b. Soap bubbles move much slower than tossed balls and balloons; the child needs the opportunity to visually follow the moving object and experience success at bursting a bubble that hovers within reach. *Occupational Therapy for Children* by Case-Smith

45. c. Adolescents want to be as independent as possible and an electric wheelchair would allow the student to arrive in class on time and preserve independence in doing so. *Occupational Therapy for Children* by Case-Smith

46. c. The goal is for the child to tie its shoes; repetition is needed in the therapy sessions as well as reinforcement at home engaging in the same task. *Hand Function in the Child* by Henderson and Pehoski

47. d. Learning to aim and direct the scissors is the next step in the hierarchy of developing scissor skills; this is best accomplished by using a straight line. *Hand Function in the Child* by Henderson and Pehoski

48. b. Only (b) makes reference to classroom behavior (sitting upright) and academic performance (written assignments). *Documentation Manual for Writing SOAP Notes in Occupational Therapy* by Borcherding

49. b. Using activity analysis, neuromuscular client factors that must be considered in bowling or other potentially strenuous activities are upper body strength, coordination to lift and maneuver the bowling ball, and endurance to carry out the activity. *Aging: The Health Care Challenge* by Lewis

50. a. Evidence is mounting that regular exercise or physical activity, such as a chair aerobic group, is a powerful tool for wellness. Many disorders can be prevented, resulting in improving the quality of life not just for the elderly but for everyone. *Functional Performance in Older Adults* by Bonder and Wagner

51. c. Most caregivers find it rewarding to continue in a role that gives them meaning; volunteering is a way to provide meaning and continue in the caregiver role. *Functional Performance in Older Adults* by Bonder and Wagner

52. c. All aging is categorized as biological, chronological, and social. *Functional Performance in Older Adults* by Bonder and Wagner

53. d. The cardiovascular system would be most stressed by lifting a weighted object while moving on an incline, such as stairs. *Functional Performance in Older Adults* by Bonder and Wagner

54. c. Clients with ulnar nerve injuries tend to claw and have weak grasps, accompanied by an inability to release. *Hand Rehabilitation: A Quick Reference Guide and Review* by Falkenstein and Weiss-Lessard

55. a. Proponents of Sensory Integration support the notion that children learn about their bodies through sensory feedback generated by movement. The exploration of an obstacle course can lead to understanding of causality and spatial relationships. This development will support the child's ability to adaptively respond to motor opportunities outside of the clinic. *Sensory Integration: Theory and Practice* by Bundy

56. b. The OT would likely recommend that the teacher avoid standing in front of the window while conducting a lesson. If the child has to look into light, such as that which comes from a window, the child will not be able to see the speaker's lips. Exaggerating mouth movements when speaking will make lip reading more difficult, as will seating the child in the back of the classroom. The teacher should talk to the child as much as other students because a hearing impaired child should receive the same amount of input as a hearing child. *Occupational Therapy for Children* by Case-Smith

57. c. The medical focus of the acute care stage after a severe burn is the replacement of lost body fluids, stabilization of the client, and care of the burn wounds. Daily wound debridement and dressing changes are needed. Occupational therapy intervention during this phase may include prevention of the loss of joint mobility, strength, and endurance. *Occupational Therapy for Children* by Case-Smith

58. d. Arthrogryposis is a condition that results in the child having stiff, spindly, and deformed joints with significantly decreased ROM. Adaptive equipment that supports independence given limited ROM, such as long-handled utensils, may assist the child in optimal functioning. *Occupational Therapy for Children* by Case-Smith

59. a. Many children with spina bifida have sensory impairments that lead to incontinence. Bowel and bladder training, or the use of a schedule that allows the child to toilet at regular intervals throughout the day, will address incontinence. The other choices are appropriate means to address toileting issues related to urgency. *Occupational Therapy for Children* by Case-Smith

60. c. Handwriting has been conceptualized as a learned motor task. In the case of handwriting, feedback is received from the pressures exerted on the writing implement and the writing surface, as well as from the senses of touch and movement in the fingers, hand, and arm and from visually monitoring the work. Feedback is used to modify and control subsequent handwriting. By allowing the child to write on a surface that provides more feedback, the OT is affording the child the opportunity to modify the amount of pressure exerted during the task. *Hand Function in the Child* by Henderson and Pehoski

61. c. A child with ADD may have to work at continuously redirecting attention from extraneous sights and sounds, as well as internal stimulation. Providing the child with a designated area to stand up and do work may help the child remain on-task and focused on the assignment. *Occupational Therapy for Children* by Case-Smith

62. a. The ulnar side of the hand offers stability so that the digits on the radial side can perform skilled movements. By encouraging the child to hold a paper clip against the palmar side of the hand with the fourth and fifth digits, the child will have to consciously flex the fingers, which will place them in a position of stability. *Hand Function in the Child* by Henderson and Pehoski

63. b. All of the mentioned professionals may be part of a feeding team. However, a pulmonary specialist would most likely have information related to the child's respiratory control. *Occupational Therapy for Children* by Case-Smith

64. b. The OT would most likely choose a global assessment that measures motor skill development in many areas. One example of such an assessment is the Peabody Developmental Motor Scales. It is a standardized assessment that would allow the OT to evaluate a child up to age 71 months on 6 subtests: reflexes, stationary, locomotion, object manipulation, grasping, and visual-motor integration. *Occupational Therapy for Children* by Case-Smith

65. a. Visual pursuit involves continuous fixation on a moving object so that the image is continuously maintained on the fovea. A child who has difficulty with visual pursuit may have difficulty with such tasks as tracking the teacher walking to a corner of the classroom. *Occupational Therapy for Children* by Case-Smith

66. c. Visual memory involves the integration of visual information with previous experiences. Adequate short-term visual memory would allow a child to hold a limited number of bits of information, such as letters and words written on a chalkboard, for approximately 30 seconds. *Occupational Therapy for Children* by Case-Smith

67. a. Clients with somatodyspraxia have difficulty planning and producing feedback-dependent movements. Verbalizing a plan can be helpful to organize movement; however, at times a child may require additional support and strategies to carry out a

complicated sequence of actions. *Sensory Integration: Theory and Practice* by Bundy

68. d. It is likely that the OT will not recommend direct service because the child is independent at school. However, the OT may recommend consultative services in order to provide the child with environmental adaptations and modifications as necessary. *Occupational Therapy for Children* by Case-Smith

69. c. An expanded keyboard would be the best choice for this student. Because of the large size of the expanded keyboard, the child with decreased fine motor control and adequate upper extremity ROM can successfully make choices on the computer. Based on the description, the child would not require a head mouse or a voice activated software program. A mini-keyboard would make the task of keyboarding more difficult for a child with poor fine motor skills, as the size of the keyboard is greatly reduced. *Pediatric Occupational Therapy and Early Intervention* by Case-Smith

70. d. The transdisciplinary approach is based on the assumption that coherence is promoted when the family primarily interacts with one or two professionals. This approach is appropriate for the infant who is medically fragile and does not tolerate multiple sources of stimulation. In this approach, all team members commit to sharing information and teaching skills to the professionals providing the direct service. *Pediatric Occupational Therapy and Early Intervention* by Case-Smith

71. d. The textured utensil would provide the child with increased sensory feedback so that the child may better be able to hold on to the utensil. *Hand Function in the Child* by Henderson and Pehoski

72. b. Using a frame will help the child to attend to one aspect of the visual field and block out the other distracting information on the page. *Occupational Therapy for Children* by Case-Smith

73. c. "Fixing" reduces the degrees of freedom at the affected joint. Fixing can lead to the shortening of muscle fibers, which can in turn lead to decreased ROM and eventually a contracture. *Frames of Reference for Pediatric Occupational Therapy* by Kramer

74. a. According to the acquisition frame of reference, providing a child with positive reinforcement or a reward for making eye contact will strengthen the response and the child will do this

more frequently. *Frames of Reference for Pediatric Occupational Therapy* by Kramer

75. b. According to the biomechanical frame of reference, in most cases a child should be positioned equally on both sides of the body. The exception is in the case of a child with scoliosis. In this case the child should be positioned so that the side of the back with the rounded part of the curvature is on the upside. Positioning in the opposite manner has the potential to exaggerate the curvature. *Handling the Young Child with Cerebral Palsy at Home* by Finnie

76. a. The use of novel and numerous activities will encourage the participation of the child who has difficulty maintaining sustained attention because it assists in retaining the child's goal-oriented attention. *Frames of Reference for Pediatric Occupational Therapy* by Kramer

77. d. The skill of holding and drinking from a bottle typically emerges around 6 months of age. *Hand Function in the Child* by Henderson and Pehoski

78. b. When working with a child during a table-top activity, such as handwriting, the table should be positioned so that it is at or slightly above elbow height. This height affords the student the opportunity to use humeral adduction with slight external rotation, which facilitates supination and wrist extension. *Hand Function in the Child* by Henderson and Pehoski

79. d. In general it is suggested that OTs encourage families to allow their children to participate in activities that naturally occur at home. Cooking activities, especially those that involve stirring, can assist in developing increased hand and arm strength. *Hand Function in the Child* by Henderson and Pehoski

80. a. The asymmetric tonic neck reflex (ATNR) is present in utero through 6–8 months while the child is awake and up to 42 months while the child is sleeping. Because of the ATNR reflex the child's head turns toward the extended arm and leg and the opposite arm and leg bend. This reflex may help in the birth process, assist in the development of visual motor integration, and protect the airway while the child is in the prone position. *Occupational Therapy in Children* by Case-Smith

81. b. Building a cube tower would also address the development of visual-motor integration skills. Hopping up and down would address the development of gross motor and bilateral

integration skills, matching a picture to an object would
address visual discrimination skills, imitating motor movements
without verbal cues would address motor planning. *Pediatric
Occupational Therapy and Early Intervention* by Case-Smith

82. c. COPD is common in children with a diagnosis of CF. If a child
was hospitalized related to complications of CF, the OT might
teach energy conservation techniques, especially those that
promote efficient breathing. A child with CF would not have
issues related to ROM, strength, or decreased balance caused by
this diagnosis. *Occupational Therapy for Children* by Case-Smith

83. a. A child with spina bifida may find a mobile stander the most
functional because the upper extremities can be used to propel
it. The mobile stander is the best choice because it promotes
the child's independence while offering an opportunity
to experience lower extremity weight bearing in standing.
Occupational Therapy for Children by Case-Smith

84. b. Transition services and goals are required as part of a student's
IEP beginning at age 14. Transition services and goals promote
the individual's movement from high school to postsecondary
life. Although goals may focus on continuing education, leisure,
and self-care, they typically involve vocational training and
community participation. *Occupational Therapy for Children* by
Case-Smith

85. c. Snipping with scissors is a prerequisite to cutting a piece of
paper in half. *Occupational Therapy for Children* by Case-Smith

86. d. This position of the paper affords the student the opportunity
to see the work while writing and prevents the smearing of
the words. The slant for a right-handed student should be
no more than 25–30 degrees to the left. The slant for a left-
handed student should be no more than 30–35 degrees to the
right. Asking the child to rest the forearms on the desk, clasp
the hands, and make the paper line up with the forearm of
the dominant hand will give a visual cue for the correct paper
placement. *Occupational Therapy for Children* by Case-Smith

87. b. By positioning the child on its side, the caregiver can be sure
that the back is extended, while making sure that the child's
arms and legs are extended as well. Carrying the child like a
baby would only reinforce the pattern of flexion. It would be
difficult to position and carry a child over the shoulder with
arms and legs extended. It is likely that in this position, the
child's neck would be hyperextended and that the child would

demonstrate excessive flexion at the shoulders. *Handling the Young Child with Cerebral Palsy at Home* by Finnie

88. b. Association is the ability to use familiar things to help recall new items. These familiar items are easy to recall and may have an emotion attached to them to aid in easy recall. Association is not used in remediation of attention, scanning, or motor planning. *Vision, Perception and Cognition* by Zoltan

89. a. According to Rood, when joint compression is greater than the person's body weight, it facilitates cocontraction at the joint undergoing the compression. If the activity was only to position in quadruped, it would be inhibitory when using normal body weight or less. This technique is not described as neutral warmth or joint compression. *Occupational Therapy Practice Skills for Physical Dysfunction* by Pedretti and Early

90. c. Positioning the body in supine is not a Bobath technique for inhibiting flexor tone. Both positioning the pelvis forward and trunk rotation techniques are used in the Bobath theory to affect overall tone, but the most effective way of helping regulate tone is through weight bearing. *Occupational Therapy Practice Skills for Physical Dysfunction* by Pedretti and Early

91. a. Although wearing clothes that utilize elastic and are larger than usual are easier, the instructions are consistent for always placing the weaker arm or leg in the garment first. *Occupational Therapy Practice Skills for Physical Dysfunction* by Pedretti and Early

92. c. Bobath theory states that ROM or movement of a subluxed shoulder should not be performed or encouraged unless the scapula is gliding and the humerus is in the proper position. *Occupational Therapy Practice Skills for Physical Dysfunction* by Pedretti and Early

93. a. Tapping is a facilitation technique described by Brunnstrom. Bobath treatment encourages the therapist's assistance of the patient through the normal movement pattern utilizing hand over hand assistance, through weight bearing, or through key points of control. Proprioceptive neuromuscular facilitation focuses on multisensory approaches and repetition to increase accuracy and speed of movement. *Occupational Therapy Practice Skills for Physical Dysfunction* by Pedretti and Early

94. c. Identifying client concerns provides the basis for knowing where to focus attention and is the foundation for generating ideas about intervention. *Willard & Spackman's Occupational Therapy,* 10th ed. by Crepeau, Cohn, and Schell

95. a. A well-stated intervention plan includes two components: the anticipated outcomes and the methods the OT and client will use to achieve those outcomes. *Willard & Spackman's Occupational Therapy,* 10th ed. by Crepeau, Cohn, and Schell

96. d. An initial short-term goal is to instruct in energy conservation and assist the patient in dealing with fatigue and pain. Because energy level and pain are more tolerable, the patient can establish a new daily routine. Creating a sense of control over the daily routine can lead to feeling of success and may have an impact on anxiety and depression. *Occupational Therapy for Physical Dysfunction* by Trombly and Radomski

97. c. Moving and static stimuli are helpful in a sensory re-education program focused on improving touch localization. Graphesthesia, the ability to identity letters and numbers traced on the skin, also is a method to improve touch localization. *Occupational Therapy for Physical Dysfunction* by Trombly and Radomski

98. d. Assessment is the OT's judgment of clients' progress, limitations, and expected benefit from therapy. *Documentation Manual for Writing SOAP Notes in Occupational Therapy by* Borcherding

99. b. Goals should be objective, functional, measurable, and action-oriented statements. *Documentation Manual for Writing SOAP Notes in Occupational Therapy* by Borcherding

100. a. The plan relates to information presented in the "O" and "A" section of the SOAP note and is a description of the interventions, methods, or approaches used to achieve the goals. *Documentation Manual for Writing SOAP Notes in Occupational Therapy* by Borcherding

101. b. When sitting at a desk, an armchair or a chair with arm rests should be used to support the upper extremities. It should allow the extremities to relax and not increase shoulder elevation, which could cause irritation to the cervicoscapular region. All items in the workstation should be within easy reach and reaching overhead should be avoided. *Upper Extremity Rehabilitation: A Practical Guide* by Burke, Higgins, McClinton, Saunders, and Valdata

102. d.   After rotator cuff surgery, gentle movement is encouraged and individuals can use the extremity as an active assist for light self-care activities, such as dressing. Persons should avoid extreme positions that may cause an increase in pain and discomfort. *Upper Extremity Rehabilitation: A Practical Guide* by Burke, Higgins, McClinton, Saunders, and Valdata

103. b.   Nonsteroidal anti-inflammatory drugs are one of the primary medications available to treat rheumatoid arthritis. These medications provide relief from pain, reduce inflammation, and are reasonable in cost. *Conditions in Occupational Therapy: Effect on Occupational Performance* by Hansen and Atchinson

104. b.   Postoperative protocol for total shoulder arthroplasty indicates that after achieving pain-free ROM to within functional limits, therapy should progress to initiation of functional activities in standing or against gravity. Activities should not be resistive in nature. *Hand and Upper Extremity Rehabilitation: A Practical Guide* by Burke, Higgins, McClinton, Saunders, and Valdata

105. c.   de Quervain's tenosynovitis is a condition characterized by localized tenderness in the first dorsal compartment of the wrist involving the extensor pollicis brevis and abductor pollicis longus tendons. Tendons may become irritated as they move around the radial styloid process. Forceful activities involving the thumb, such as pinch, usually exacerbate the pain and discomfort. *Hand and Upper Extremity Rehabilitation: A Practical Guide* by Burke, Higgins, McClinton, Saunders, and Valdata

106. d.   Rhythmic games and activities are beneficial for persons with Parkinson's disease, particularly in terms of improving motor skills. *Occupational Therapy Practice Skills for Physical Dysfunction* by Pedretti and Early

107. c.   A stand pivot transfer is an assisted transfer that is used when a person has lower extremity weakness but is able to put some weight on one or both legs. *Occupational Therapy for Physical Dysfunction* by Trombly and Radomski

108. c.   To prevent back injury with transfers, the person performing the technique should keep the back and spine as straight as possible and lift or rotate using the strong arm muscles. *Occupational Therapy for Physical Dysfunction* by Trombly and Radomski

109. a.   Principles of work simplification support planning ahead and creating a schedule to distribute energy demanding tasks

throughout the week, prioritizing the most importance tasks before fatiguing. *Occupational Therapy for Physical Dysfunction* by Trombly and Radomski

110. c.   A general model for learning compensatory cognitive strategies includes four phases: (1) anticipation—learning about and gaining insight into the consequences of cognitive deficits; (2) acquisition—learning compensatory strategies to deal with cognitive deficits through practice; (3) application—using compensatory strategies during simulated and real-life activities; and (4) adaptation—adapting strategies to additional areas of occupation. *Occupational Therapy for Physical Dysfunction* by Trombly and Radomski

111. d.   Clothes that contribute to independence in dressing would be front opening, loose fitting garments with large fasteners or Velcro closures. *Occupational Therapy for Physical Dysfunction* by Trombly and Radomski

112. b.   Goals should be realistic, measurable, and have element of function with specific condition(s) and/or time frame. *Documentation manual for Writing SOAP Notes in Occupational Therapy* by Borcherding

113. c.   Environments that use universal designs are adaptable, accessible, generally low cost, aesthetically pleasing, and can be used by a wide range of people with various needs throughout much of the lifespan. *Occupational Therapy for Physical Dysfunction* by Trombly and Radomski

114. d.   After learning to visually attend to stimuli, the next step is to do visual tracking in different planes, such as horizontal and vertical. *Occupational Therapy for Physical Dysfunction* by Trombly and Radomski

115. c.   Principle 3 of the Code of Ethics deals with autonomy and respecting the rights of the client. Furthermore, practitioners should collaborate with recipients, families, significant others, and/or caregivers in setting goals and priorities throughout the intervention process. *AOTA: Code of Ethics Document*

116. a.   Inpatient cardiac rehabilitation has several goals including preventing muscle atrophy while on bed rest, assessing and monitoring functional abilities, and educating the individual on risk factors and appropriate home activities for discharge. *Occupational Therapy for Physical Dysfunction* by Trombly and Radomski

117. a. Games, crafts, and self-care tasks are functional tasks that are helpful for improving hand rehabilitation. *Hand and Upper Extremity Rehabilitation* by Burke, Higgins, McClinton, Saunders and Valdata

118. c. Under Medicare, "medically necessary" means the equipment is primarily and customarily used by the individual during the course of the illness or condition. *The Occupational Therapy Manager* by McCormack, Jaffe, and Goodman-Lavey

119. c. Isometric exercises are contraindicated for person with cardiovascular problems because blood pressure and heart rate may increase. *Occupational Therapy Practice Skills for Physical Dysfunction* by Pedretti and Early

120. d. The problem list should include the underlying factor that is causing the performance deficit. *Documentation Manual for Writing SOAP Notes in Occupational Therapy* by Borcherding

121. d. According to the Model of Human Occupation, it is important to comprehend the influence and interaction of both personal and environmental elements. An evaluation would focus on the effect of personal traits and the environment on role performance. *Occupational Therapy in Community-Based Practice Setting* by Scaffa

122. d. The term pragmatic reasoning is a type of clinical reasoning that addresses the practical context and personal context. This includes treatment resources, organizational climate, reimbursement issues, and practice trends in the profession. *Willard & Spackman's Occupational Therapy,* 10th ed. by Crepeau, Cohn, and Schell

123. c. Maximum assistance is defined as providing verbal cueing and/or physical assistance approximately 50%–75% of the time a person is performing a task. *Occupational Therapy Practice Skills for Physical Dysfunction* by Pedretti and Early

124. c. With TBI, there are several levels of cognitive functioning including no response, confused-agitated, confused with inappropriate behaviors, confused with appropriate behaviors, automatic-appropriate, and purposeful-appropriate. For a person with confusion but appropriate behaviors, the focus should be on providing cues and direction for self-care tasks, and minimal supervision for safety is usually required. *Quick Reference to Occupational Therapy* by Reed

125. b. There are several levels of cognitive functioning in persons who experience a TBI, including no response, confused-agitated, confused with inappropriate behaviors, confused with appropriate behaviors, automatic-appropriate, and purposeful-appropriate. For a person with confusion and agitation, low-level interventions should be used related to attention span, memory, and safety. *Quick Reference to Occupational Therapy* by Reed

126. d. The cognitive behavioral model would address both cognitive issues and behavioral outbursts. The goal of intervention is to provide a safe environment that enables the individual to be further assessed and participate in a comprehensive program. *Quick Reference to Occupational Therapy* by Reed

127. c. Patients with osteoporosis should receive instructions in safety procedures including the use of grab bars, handrails, elimination of floor hazards, and use good lighting. They should also follow principles of joint protection to minimize chances of injury. *Quick Reference to Occupational Therapy* by Reed

128. b. Using visual cues combined with auditory input will provide dual means of addressing the issue of auditory processing. Visual cues will reinforce the auditory input. *Quick Reference to Occupational Therapy* by Reed

129. c. Answers (a) and (b) are not appropriate to the patient's immediate needs at this time, and (d) is not a complete and measurable goal. *Mental Health Concepts and Techniques for the Occupational Therapy Assistant* by Early

130. d. Tact is crucial in such a situation and it is important for the OT to take every opportunity to educate new physicians and build solid relationships. Any intervention provided must follow the physician's orders, so it is crucial that the order be written appropriately. *Mental Health Concepts and Techniques for the Occupational Therapy Assistant* by Early

131. d. Before an OT can intervene to encourage participation, they must understand what is causing the person to refuse. This knowledge may allow the therapist to make adaptations that support participation. *Mental Health Concepts and Techniques for the Occupational Therapy Assistant* by Early

132. a. Despite the fact that venting feelings might be beneficial, it is most important, from a developmental approach, to concretely build the necessary skills to function effectively in

age-appropriate occupations with peers. *Group Dynamics in Occupational Therapy* by Cole

133. a. Getting active is important for the client and increasing socialization opportunities might help as well. Option (a) addresses these issues in a measurable format. *Proactive Approaches in Psychosocial Occupational Therapy* by Fleming

134. c. The student will use a visual schedule to independently transition between class activities, 80% of the time, by end of the semester. Educational goals should reflect outcomes of the curriculum and educational priorities of the child. *Occupational Therapy for Children* by Case-Smith

135. d. Children may be ready for formal handwriting instruction when they have mastered the first 9 designs on the Developmental Test of Visual Motor Integration. *Occupational Therapy for Children* by Case-Smith

136. c. Children snip with scissors at age 2, cut across a page by 2.5 years, cut on a line by 3 to 3.5 years, cut a circle by 3.5 to 4 years, and cut a square by 4.5 to 5 years. *Occupational Therapy for Children* by Case-Smith

137. c. Following identification of an educational problem, the IEP team determines the need for school-based occupational therapy services. *OT Services for Children and Youth Under the IDEA*, AOTA

138. a. Following identification of an educational problem, the IEP team determines the need for school-based occupational therapy services. *OT Services for Children and Youth Under the IDEA*, AOTA

139. c. A sensory diet contains a few activity suggestions effective for an individual to meet specific needs throughout the day. Once developed by a qualified therapist, it can be applied by caregivers into daily lives. *Sensory Integration I Theory and Practice* by Bundy

140. d. A notebook sent back and forth between home and school allows daily exchange of information including progress, concerns, and new strategies. *Occupational Therapy for Children* by Case-Smith

141. d. Occupational therapy goals in the school system reflect educational outcomes. *AOTA: Applying Sensory Integration*

Framework in Educationally Related Occupational Therapy Practice

142. c. The OT selects the appropriate frame of reference based on the evaluation using clinical reasoning. *AOTA Statement: Applying Sensory Integration Framework in Educationally Related Occupational Therapy Practice*

143. a. The child is seeking deep pressure and is using the side of the bed for this input.

144. d. A patient with arthritis needs to strike a balance between activity and rest. The more inflammation, the more rest is required and less exercise and vise versa. Excessive movement can aggravate inflammation and lack of movement may increase stiffness. *Basic Rehabilitation Techniques: A Self Instructional Guide* by Sine, Liss, Roush, Holcomb, and Wilson

CHAPTER 6

Questions for Intervention

Intervention is the process of facilitating changes in the occupation and performance skills of a client. Intervention consists of putting a plan into action that modifies performance deficits and positively impacts the client factors, roles, habits, and routines that are valued by the recipient. Outcomes of intervention are restoration of skills that are meaningful, optimization of functional abilities, implementation of new skills, and compensation for the loss of function.

1. The Individualized Family Service Plan (IFSP) is established in early intervention by the:
   a. Assessment team without family input
   b. Assessment team with family input
   c. Family without team input
   d. Primary therapy service

2. An occupational therapist (OT) has begun implementing intervention strategies with an infant. One of the parents is very anxious about making sure that the strategies that the OT is utilizing are followed correctly. The BEST method for teaching the parent the strategies is:
   a. To provide written handouts
   b. To model techniques in sessions
   c. To gear to parent learning style
   d. To provide illustrations and videos

3. An OT arrives at a child's home to begin a treatment session. When the therapist enters the home the child is running through the house screeching. The OT determines that the FIRST step in the intervention session will be:
   a. Sitting still on a therapy ball
   b. Placing the child in a high chair
   c. Rhythmic linear swinging
   d. Rapidly brushing extremities

4. A goal of early intervention is to provide family-centered service. When an OT assists families in having a clearer understanding of their child's disabilities and strengths, it is an example of:
    a. Compensation
    b. Adaptation
    c. Supporting
    d. Reframing

5. An OT in early intervention suggests to a family that their child, who is sensory defensive, would benefit from having the tags cut out of his T-shirts. The term that BEST describes this type of intervention is:
    a. Adaptation
    b. Supportive
    c. Reframing
    d. Remediation

6. A child being treated in occupational therapy cries and becomes upset whenever it is touched lightly or unexpectedly. The OT recommends to the child's parents that the child should be touched using deep pressure. This is an example of utilizing techniques for:
    a. Sensory discrimination
    b. Sensory modulation
    c. Vestibular receptivity
    d. Tactile responsivity

7. A child has transitioned from early intervention into preschool. The child has Asperger's disorder and attention deficit hyperactivity disorder (ADHD). The child has problems sitting still for more than 5 minutes during class. The teacher has contacted the school OT to find out how to help this child. The therapist recommends that the BEST way to address this issue is:
    a. Put the child in time out in a quiet place
    b. Allow the child to bounce on a therapy ball
    c. Redirect the child to sit and complete the activity
    d. Have the child stand while up against a wall

8. A child has poor ability to maintain trunk and neck extension. The OT uses which of the following as the BEST technique to facilitate increased strength and control:
    a. Have child prone on a therapy ball and play with toys
    b. Have child supine on a platform swing while playing with toys
    c. Have child in side lying on a mat shield playing with toys
    d. Have child sit on physioball while playing with toys

9. An OT working with a 2-month-old child alternates between repeatedly raising the child from a supine position into sitting and slowly lowering the child back into a supine position. The OT is MOST likely trying to elicit:
   a. Protective reactions
   b. Neck lateralization
   c. Neck flexion
   d. Reflex reactions

10. An OT is working with a child who has cerebral palsy. The child has limited range of motion (ROM) in bilateral upper extremities and is unable to reach out for objects. The OT provides intervention that focuses on allowing the child to participate in play activities. The BEST position to place the child in is:
    a. Sidelying
    b. Prone
    c. Supine
    d. Sitting

11. A child has difficulty searching for objects that have dropped from the wheelchair tray. The BEST method for the OT to use to adapt the child's environment so the child can engage in play and foster independence is to:
    a. Have the child play when someone is present
    b. Have the child watch videos
    c. Tie a string to toys that is attached to the wheelchair
    d. Lower the tray and place at a slight angle

12. A child has difficulty with in-hand manipulation or only finger to palm transition to manipulate objects between two hands, and uses support surfaces to assist in object manipulation. The therapist can use which of the following activities to improve this occupational performance:
    a. Surfaces as a support
    b. Objects that roll
    c. Tiny objects
    d. Hold hands away

13. A child is participating in sensory integrative therapy. During the intervention session, the OT notices that the child does NOT become dizzy during a spinning activity. The OT discusses this with the child's mother and explains that the child is:
    a. Hyperresponsive
    b. Hyporesponsive
    c. Sensory defensive
    d. Gravitationally insecure

14. A second grader with cerebral palsy has demonstrated poor handwriting skills. The child has difficulty holding a pencil and very restricted hand movement. The child is an average student and does not appear to have any cognitive learning disabilities. A recommendation for the intervention plan for second grade, based on her needs in fourth and fifth grade, would be:
    a. Begin to teach the child keyboarding skills to prepare for word processing using a computer for written assignments
    b. Provide systemic practice using kinesthetic patterns to improve letter formation and legibility
    c. Use templates for alphabets so that the child can practice and learn letter formation
    d. Enforce a strict writing program in the classroom for the teacher to implement

15. An effective compensatory strategy that can be used with children is:
    a. Providing deep pressure using a weighted vest to a child with hypersensitivities
    b. Praising a child when sharing his materials with a peer
    c. Providing peel-off stickers to a child who has poor drawing skills
    d. Having the child sit on a physioball during art class

16. A child has difficulty coordinating two hands together. The child tends to neglect his left hand. To provide more proprioceptive input to the child's left arm and to strengthen it, you design a bilateral activity in which the child wears a 2-pound weight on the left wrist. This type of intervention strategy is:
    a. Grading the activity to provide the "just right" challenge
    b. Modifying the environment
    c. Promoting participation and preventing disability
    d. Providing augmented sensory cueing and feedback

17. A type of sensory input that has a strong effect on arousal that is used by OTs to prepare a child for a therapeutic activity is:
    a. Vestibular input by swinging the child
    b. Visual input through a computer game
    c. Olfactory input with harsh odors
    d. Auditory input by reading the child a story

18. A child with ADHD and sensory modulation dysfunction is being treated in occupational therapy using a sensory integrative approach. An intervention strategy that is used to improve his ability to attend in the classroom would be:
    a. Using occupation as means
    b. Modifying the environment

    c. Therapeutic use of self

    d. Group work

19. The BEST statement regarding the use of Neurodevelopmental Treatment (NDT) with children is:

    a. NDT is most effective for certain children, primarily those with cerebral palsy, in developing specific motor skills.

    b. Performance areas targeted when using NDT should not be specifically and routinely measured to determine whether progress toward expected outcomes is satisfactory.

    c. Clinical trials have demonstrated that functional performance in children who receive intensive NDT is significantly higher than the performance of children who receive regular occupational therapy that emphasized functional activities.

    d. Clinical trials have demonstrated that NDT is effective for infants with spastic diplegia.

20. OTs contribute to the goal of inclusion for all children. When children are included, services are provided in a:

    a. Natural environment

    b. Special education classroom

    c. Specifically designated area

    d. Rehabilitation clinic

21. Evidence-based practice is the determination of intervention strategies based on:

    a. Extant research findings

    b. Research findings, the OT's own experiences, and family priorities

    c. An OT's expert opinion

    d. Other disciplines' practice

22. An important cultural consideration when working with a child with behavioral issues and the family is:

    a. The family's view of disability

    b. A therapist's personal views

    c. Societal views of the family's culture

    d. Societal expectations of the disabled

23. A way to distinguish an Interdisciplinary Model from a Multidisciplinary Model is:

    a. The team requires group synthesis

    b. Members always have consensus

    c. Each member is respected for his or her expertise in a defined practice area

    d. Members have a good understanding of other professionals' scopes of practice

24. Which of the following services for children are primarily provided by physical therapists?
    a. Motor learning
    b. Fine motor
    c. Augmentative communication
    d. Social skill development

25. An early intervention service listed in Part C of the Individuals with Education Act (IDEA) is:
    a. Prenatal care
    b. Medical care and surgery
    c. Music therapy
    d. Nutrition

26. An interdisciplinary team is working with a fourth-grade student who receives special education and related services and is demonstrating problem behaviors. The FIRST step the team should follow is:
    a. Develop a comprehensive description of the problem, including individual and environmental factors that influence the issue
    b. Make a decision and develop a plan for achieving the solution
    c. Define the roles the multiple services have been playing in the child's intervention plan
    d. Identify as many strategies as possible to reduce barriers and increase supports

27. What role do nurses play in early intervention for children?
    a. Providing educational materials on augmentative communication and mobility equipment
    b. Screening and assessing the psychologic, physiologic, and developmental characteristics of the child and family
    c. Providing treatment to increase joint function, muscle strength, mobility, and endurance
    d. Provide social skills training for the child as is appropriate

28. A medically fragile preterm infant was recently discharged from the hospital. His early intervention team provides home-based services using a transdisciplinary model with the nurse as the primary interventionist. The intervention provided by the OT on this team would be:
    a. Consulting with and coaching the nurse
    b. Providing one-on-one intervention in the home
    c. Assisting with group sessions in the clinic
    d. Co-treating with other therapy services in the clinic

29. An 8-year-old child with normal intelligence has trouble
     concentrating on schoolwork. The social worker reveals to the
     OT that one of the child's parents has been unemployed for some
     time, while the other parent does odd jobs to make ends meet. In
     reflecting on these issues and Maslow's hierarchy of needs, the OT
     might conclude that:
     a. The child is acting out against their parents because of their
         living situation
     b. The child is probably borderline learning disability
     c. Basic physiological needs of the child are not being met
     d. Basic safety needs of the child are not being met

30. A 6-year-old has some difficulty taking part in group activities with
     friends at school. An explanation of this child's behavior using the
     dynamic systems approach would be:
     a. Learns and develops certain skills by observing the behavior of
         others
     b. Functional performance would depend on the interactions of
         the child's inherent and emerging skills, the characteristics of
         the desired task or activity, and the environment in which the
         activity is performed
     c. Develops a system by which to extract information from the
         environment and interpret the information
     d. Organizes a behavioral response such as a motor skill

31. A 6-year-old has gaps in handwriting skills that can improve
     with an intensive, repetitive program that focuses on acquisition
     or learning of these skills. A behavior that the child would
     exhibit during this stage of intervention to improve handwriting
     would be:
     a. At the acquisition stage, a child observes the behavior of others
         and determines the consequences, and these observations are
         stored in memory for later use.
     b. The child may decide to perform the behavior, depending
         on the child's perception of the situation and the
         consequences.
     c. Children first experience activities (e.g., problem solving)
         in situations in which a child, an activity, and an adult are
         components and then gradually the adult's speech becomes part
         of the child's cognitive repertoire.
     d. The child is guided only by an adult during activities.

32. An 8-year-old with sensory processing problems has been referred to
     the school-based OT. The child is sensory-seeking and active in the
     classroom by hitting and biting other children. The child does not seem
     aware that these behaviors are socially inappropriate. Deep pressure

helps the child focus up to at least 10 minutes. The BEST method from the coping model to assist the child with coping and developing peer relations in the classroom would be:

a. Allow the child unsupervised interaction with their peers, where they feels less pressured and would likely develop peer relations with students in the second-grade classroom

b. Reorganize material and people around the child to allow the child to focus better on the activity at hand. Personal social skills may be emphasized by practice of social skills in the context of games with peers. Timely, positive, and explicit feedback to the child's coping efforts helps the child experience a sense of mastery.

c. Create an environment for artistic development by providing the child with colors, paper, clay, and toys that bring out the child's creativity

d. Provide bouncing on a physioball and swinging from a platform covered with cushioning

33. An appropriate sensorimotor activity for an infant of age up to 6 months is:

a. Sitting erect and unsupported for several minutes
b. Rolling sequentially to progress across the room
c. Crawling forward
d. Pulling to stand

34. The grasp a 5-year-old child uses to firmly hold a pencil to write or draw is a:

a. Static tripod grasp
b. Dynamic tripod grasp
c. Pincer grasp
d. Radial digital grasp

35. An OT is treating a 4-year-old child who has demonstrated delays in reaching major motor milestones. The child's parents ask if their child will be able to attend a regular school and live a normal healthy life in the future. A response the OT can provide to address their concerns is:

a. Make definitive optimistic statements about the future to boost their morale

b. Tell them that it's not possible to make any predictions about the future

c. Help parents understand the range of possibilities by telling them about the continuum of services for older children and young adults in the community

d. Tell them that the future outlook for their child is bleak

36. A 2-year-old toddler has delays in communication, play, and self-feeding. The child's parents have moderate mental retardation

and both of them work from home to earn their daily living.
A strategy that the OT could suggest to help them in working with their child is:

a. Disregard their limited problem-solving skills
b. Make decisions for them when they have difficulty planning the next step
c. Ignore their internal and external control, self-esteem, and social skills
d. Take note of their learning styles and abilities so as to better instruct them

37. A 5-year-old has special needs that make it difficult for the child to participate in community activities with other children. The child's parents are concerned that they are the only socialization agents for the child, because community social activities simply do not accommodate their child. Most social interactions are with adults, and the child has never really interacted with peers or made friends. This is a source of great stress for the parents. A coping strategy that the OT could suggest is:

a. Participate in recreational and leisure activities that will expose the child to environments other than the house or school
b. Develop friendships with other parents in a similar situation and form part of a support group
c. Discuss alternative strategies with the OT that will help the child perform daily living activities with greater skill and independence
d. Discuss with the OT the various professional services that are available

38. A 4½-year-old child is diagnosed with dyskinetic cerebral palsy. The OT treating the child needs to assess the child in order to design an appropriate intervention program. Which of the following standardized tests should the OT administer?

a. School Function Assessment (SFA)
b. Gross Motor Function Measure (GMFM)
c. Sensory Integration and Praxis Tests (SIPT)
d. Miller Assessment for Preschoolers (MAP)

39. A 2-year-old child shows poor head control in the prone and sitting positions. What intervention would the OT to motivate and help the child gain head control?

a. Use of a therapeutic ball
b. Use of a therapeutic wedge
c. Biofeedback
d. Use of toys or the parent's voice to motivate the child

40. The OT working with a child on motor disabilities could not see any progress. In analyzing the intervention, it was noticed that the OT gave frequent feedback to the child at each step. The OT made the child frequently repeat the movements and also held the child's hands while doing the movements in practice sessions. In spite of the OT's efforts, there was no progress in the child's motor learning. Which of the following do you think are the reasons for the child's failure?
    a. Random scheduling
    b. Need more feedback
    c. Require more repetition of movements over a long period of time
    d. Handling may cause ineffective motor learning

41. A 5-year-old child exhibits left spastic hemiplegia, associated increased tone, forearm pronation, and fisting during stressful activities. With the left hand, the child is able to use a palmar grasp and rarely uses this hand as a stabilizer in bilateral activities. The child also has difficulty completing in-hand manipulation activities with the right hand as the only in-hand manipulation skills, but is able to consistently use finger to palm translation and palm to finger translation. Which of the following types of hand skill activities are MOST likely to be appropriate for intervention at this time?
    a. Pincer grasp with the left hand
    b. Stabilization of objects with grasp with the left hand
    c. Complex rotation with stabilization skills
    d. Simultaneous bilateral manipulation skills

42. Which of the following is a key precaution in using hand splinting for children with spasticity?
    a. The splint should not be worn during the day, in order to allow for hand use
    b. The splint should not be worn at night if there is hand flexion during sleep
    c. The child should wear a splint initially for at least 6–8 hours per day
    d. The therapist should see the child frequently for follow-up intervention

43. Which of the following theories/approaches would be MOST associated with intervention emphasizing structure and feedback during performance of a hand skill as well as repetition of the activities?
    a. Motor learning theory
    b. Developmental frame of reference
    c. Sensory integration frame of reference
    d. Behavioral theory

44. A 4-year-old preschooler has difficulty building with LEGO blocks because of the use of an immature pincer grasp, poor voluntary release skills, and difficulty stabilizing objects with one hand while manipulating with the other. Which of the following is MOST likely to be one of the intervention strategies that the OT would use?
    a. Promote the child's ability to vary all joint positions in the arm while sustaining grasp
    b. Provide splinting to support the wrist
    c. Emphasize development of a mature finger pad grasp pattern
    d. Improve symmetrical bilateral hand skills

45. Which of the following intervention strategies would you choose to use with children who possess basic in-hand manipulation skills but need to improve them?
    a. Encourage the child to manipulate objects between the two hands
    b. Provide verbal cueing and/or demonstration of skills
    c. Use materials to promote complex rotation with stabilization skills
    d. Use support surfaces to assist in object manipulation

46. Which of the following are characteristics of classic sensory integration treatment?
    a. It can be applied individually or in groups
    b. It is given in the form of consultation
    c. It puts emphasis on the inner drive of the child
    d. It uses group therapy programs

47. An 18-month-old was diagnosed with sensory integration dysfunction. The child is undergoing occupational therapy as well as speech therapy for speech delays. The child's parents are eager to know the length of time required to cure their child. How would an OT address their concern?
    a. Give them a tentative time period based on the severity of the problem
    b. Tell them that occupational therapy aims at improving the sensory integrative functions and the quality of life of a child
    c. Tell them that it is impossible to give a fixed time period
    d. Tell them the child will never be cured

48. A 5-year-old displays disorganized behavior. The child's mother says that the child is not spontaneous during play or school activities. For example, the child has trouble completing a simple puzzle and when left alone wanders aimlessly. The child's peers say the child is slow. Which of the following BEST describes such behavior?
    a. He is clumsy and awkward.
    b. He has dyspraxia.
    c. He has somatodyspraxia.
    d. He has difficulty in bilateral integration and sequencing.

49. A client diagnosed with a wrist sprain is referred to occupational therapy for a splint to promote rest but also to allow hand use. The OT would most likely fabricate a splint so that the:
    a. Hand is posed in a functional position
    b. Palmar bar is proximal to the distal palmar crease
    c. Palmar bar is distal to the distal palmar crease
    d. Width is less than one-half the circumference of the forearm

50. A patient with a diagnosis of arthritis was referred for splinting to alleviate symptoms of pain and swelling in the distal right upper extremity. Which splint design would be the MOST appropriate?
    a. A resting hand splint
    b. A static progressive splint
    c. A dynamic splint
    d. A serial static cast

51 An elderly patient exhibits skin breakdown caused by perspiration while wearing a splint. The OT would MOST likely correct this problem by addressing:
    a. Conformability of the splint
    b. Elasticity of the splint
    c. Permeability of the splint
    d. Drapability of the splint

52. A child diagnosed with cerebral palsy has severe spasticity in the bilateral upper extremities. The occupational therapy referral states "fabricate splints to prevent hand deformities." The theoretical approach for splinting should emphasize placement of the hands in the:
    a. Intrinsic minus position
    b. Anticlaw position
    c. Resting hand position
    d. Reflex inhibiting position

53. A client with rheumatoid arthritis has developed a boutonniere deformity of the right index finger. In order to correct this deformity, the OT must fabricate a splint that positions the:
    a. Proximal interphalangeal joint into extension and the distal interphalangeal joint into flexion
    b. Proximal interphalangeal joint and the distal interphalangeal joint into flexion
    c. Proximal interphalangeal joint into hyperextension and the distal interphalangeal joint into flexion
    d. Metacarpal in flexion and the proximal interphalangeal joint and the distal interphalangeal joint into extension

54. The OT is treating a patient in the acute care burn unit who recently experienced deep partial thickness burns to the left upper and lower extremities. The main focus of splinting is:
    a. Scar reduction and management
    b. To prevent the spread of infection
    c. Joint mobility as the wound heals
    d. Functional use of the upper extremity

55. A 50-year-old patient with a crush injury to the right dominant hand has severe pitting edema. The BEST technique for the OT to use for splinting is:
    a. To provide a standard resting hand splint that promotes finger-thumb opposition
    b. To place extremity in a functional position and use a wide bandage to hold splint in place
    c. To use a dynamic splint that allows periodic controlled motion of the involved extremity
    d. To provide an antispasticity hand splint and use wide straps to hold splint in place

56. An elderly patient with carpal tunnel syndrome was provided a dorsal-based wrist cock-up splint 1 week earlier. During the next visit, the patient complained of pain and discomfort over the radial styloid area after wearing the splint for 60 minutes. The OT should:
    a. Place padding inside the splint over the affected area
    b. Discard the splint and fabricate another
    c. Spot heat the splint and stretch out over the affected area
    d. Decrease the amount of splint wear time to 30 minutes

57. A patient with recent hip replacement surgery was advised to continue to follow hip precautions when discharged home. An important piece of adaptive equipment that the OT might recommend is:
    a. A wheelchair
    b. Velcro shoes
    c. A sliding board
    d. A raised toilet seat

58. Which activity of daily living (ADL) activity would the OT caution a patient with a recent hip replacement to avoid?
    a. Tying shoes
    b. Pulling up pants
    c. Putting on shirt
    d. Bathing the back

59. A patient with a T1 spinal cord injury wants to become independent in functional mobility. The OT should incorporate:
    a. Teaching the patient how to use a manual wheelchair
    b. Walking using short leg braces and crutches
    c. Drivers training in a regular vehicle
    d. Caregiver's training to assist the patient with mobility

60. During a treatment session, a patient with a C5 spinal cord injury complains of dizziness and a severe headache and is noticed by the OT to be flushed and sweating profusely. The BEST course of action for the OT to take is to:
    a. Lie the patient down to rest for about 30 minutes or until symptoms subside
    b. Contact the physician and report signs of autonomic dysreflexia
    c. Take the blood pressure because of the suspected signs of orthostatic hypotension
    d. Assist the patient in taking medication for the symptoms

61. A 30-year-old patient sustains an isolated, minimally displaced fracture of the left wrist as a result of a fall. The initial treatment includes immobilization in a dorsal splint secured with an Ace bandage and the extremity positioned in a sling. The NEXT step in treatment should consist of:
    a. Activities related to strengthening
    b. Application of the splint for an additional 10 days
    c. Controlled active mobilization
    d. Application of a hinged elbow splint

62. A client with a right cerebrovascular accident (CVA) has a severe flexor synergy pattern of the left upper extremity. What type of splint should the OT recommend to promote functional movement and engagement in occupation?
    a. Resting hand
    b. Wrist cock-up
    c. Anti-spasticity
    d. Ulnar gutter

63. A client with a 1-week-old crush injury of the right hand caused by a factory accident is referred for splinting. The injury resulted in a loss of muscle tissue in the hand and the wound has not completely healed. To facilitate healing and function, the optimal splinting position that the OT should use is the:
    a. Resting hand position
    b. Intrinsic plus
    c. Intrinsic minus
    d. Hand in full extension

64. A patient with intention tremors is observed to have frequent spills of food and drink while eating. To facilitate greater control during mealtime, the OT should:
   a. Provide a large, long-handled tablespoon for eating
   b. Use a weighted cuff on the wrist to assist patient during meals
   c. Train a caregiver to assist the patient during meals
   d. Raise the eating surface closer to the face

65. A child with a diagnosis of ADHD has considerable difficulty paying attention in school and also has difficulty with coordination. Which activity would be the MOST effective intervention to promote learning for this child?
   a. Assembling a colorful puzzle with two other students
   b. Playing a rhythmic clapping game about numbers
   c. Blowing bubbles with other students on the playground
   d. Removing the child from the rest of classmates to work alone

66. A child who is blind is tactilely defensive. The child recently started kindergarten, and the OT is asked to recommend a method to assist the child to learn Braille. The BEST method for initiating treatment with this child is to:
   a. Play games that involve following an obstacle course over various textures
   b. Lightly stroke the child's arms and legs with various textures
   c. Play seek and find with cotton balls within the child's reach
   d. Use several scratch and sniff activities during play

67. An OT would recommend the use of a wheelchair with removable arms to a client with:
   a. A head injury who gets confused when trying to use the arm rests
   b. Ataxia who needs to use the bathroom sink
   c. A T4 spinal cord lesion performing transfers
   d. Alzheimer's who has difficulty reaching items on the floor

68. A 7-year-old child exhibits problems with gravitational insecurity. The BEST playground activity the OT can recommend to the parent is to have the child to:
   a. Hang upside down on the jungle gym
   b. Play on the sliding board
   c. Roll in the sandbox
   d. Play on the swing set

69. An OT works in an early intervention program with children that exhibit sensory integration deficits. The BEST approach to improve the children's sensory deficits and occupational performance is to:
   a. Promote random play activities

   b. Promote activities that facilitate equilibrium and righting reactions

   c. Provide controlled motor, proprioceptive, and tactile activities

   d. Provide group activities that increase interactive play

70. A patient with arthritis has a boutonniere deformity of the left middle finger. To correct the deformity, the OT would position the digit in:

   a. PIP joint extension and DIP joint hyperextension

   b. PIP joint extension and DIP extension

   c. Both PIP and DIP joint flexion

   d. PIP flexion and DIP

71. The OT is working on feeding with a child who is hypertonic. The BEST method to use for jaw control while feeding is to:

   a. Apply hand to child's chin from front or side to promote chin tuck and provide stability to jaw

   b. Apply one hand to forehead and the other hand to chin to control opening and closing of the mouth

   c. Apply pressure to sides of jaw at the mouth level and press to facilitate opening of the mouth

   d. Apply hand to forehead and push head into extension to facilitate opening of the mouth

72. An elderly homemaker underwent a total hip replacement 7 days ago. The patient is being discharged with a home program. Following hip precautions, the OT should recommend that when performing some basic ADL tasks, the patient should avoid:

   a. Leaning over a counter right in front to reach into cabinets

   b. Bathing in the shower

   c. Picking up pants from the floor with a reacher

   d. Sitting on a regular toilet

73. A patient in a chronic pain management program exhibits constant complaining negative behavior about the presence and intensity of pain. One approach to assist in extinguishing the constant complaining is to:

   a. Sympathize with the patient when he or she complains

   b. Refer the patient to the physician or nurse for medication

   c. Confront the patient about the constant complaining

   d. Ignore the constant complaining and focus on the positive when it occurs

74. A technique that an OT working with a patient with a C5 spinal cord injury would recommend is:

   a. Perform wheelchair push ups

b. Rely on a caregiver
c. Shift weight by using arm rests
d. Use a gel cushion

75. A patient with a long-term illness has been bedridden for longer than a month. The condition of the patient has improved. The patient can now perform bed mobility and transfer in and out of bed into a chair for basic self-care without fatigue. Using a progressive mobilization program to improve occupational performance, the NEXT step for the home health OT is to:
a. Extend the time for performing ADL tasks in sitting
b. Move to the bathroom for performing ADLs
c. Add additional tasks to be performed at bedside
d. Begin performing some ADL tasks in standing while at bedside

76. A patient diagnosed with arthritis complains of pain in the elbows and forearm and has difficulty with self-feeding. ROM assessment reveals limitation in pronation and supination, but elbow flexion and extension are within functional limits. The BEST piece of adapted equipment to use for independence in self-feeding is:
a. Long-handled lightweight utensils
b. Built-up handled utensils
c. Utensils placed in a universal cuff
d. A swivel spoon or fork

77. A patient with rheumatoid arthritis complains of pain in bilateral shoulders when reaching overhead and performing cooking activities. ROM measurements reveal approximately 80 –83 degrees of active ROM in shoulders and 100–110 degrees of PROM. Using an adapted technique, the OT should recommend:
a. Standing to perform cooking and to obtain items overhead
b. Incorporating active ROM and passive stretching
c. Using a long-handled lightweight piece of adapted equipment
d. Using a reacher

78. An OT is working in a rehabilitation setting with an individual who has emphysema and is dependent on oxygen. While providing intervention to improve home management, the OT should:
a. Monitor activity tolerance using a pulse oximeter
b. Limit activity until oxygen is discontinued
c. Request oxygen be discontinued during activities
d. Keep treatment session short no more than 15 minutes

79. An OT is working with an individual who has low back pain and works as a truck driver. Using the biomechanical approach the OT should:
a. Assess the individual to determine other job options

b. Recommend the person consider part-time work until pain diminishes

c. Refer the person to physical therapy or a chiropractor

d. Educate on proper positioning for the work environment

80. A medically fragile preterm infant was recently discharged from the neonatal unit at the hospital. The early intervention team has set up home-based services using a transdisciplinary model with the nurse as the primary interventionist. Using this model, the OT's service for the infant is to:
    a. Provide a home program for the family
    b. Provide one-on-one intervention in the home
    c. Assist with group sessions in the clinic
    d. Consult with and coaches the nurse

81. A schoolteacher requests the assistance of the OT to recommend activities to facilitate drawing in a 4-year-old child. The OT would advise the teacher that an appropriate activity to facilitate drawing is to have the student:
    a. Draw circles and lines
    b. Imitate simple figures
    c. Connect the dots
    d. Play tic tac toe

82. A 5-year-old child has mastered a pincer grasp for writing in school. In order to progress, the OT should provide writing activities to facilitate a:
    a. Primitive pincer grasp
    b. Dynamic tripod grasp
    c. Palmar grasp
    d. Radial digital grasp

83. A 2-year-old child with cerebral palsy has poor head control in the prone and sitting positions. One technique to engage the child and facilitate head control is:
    a. Using of a therapeutic ball
    b. Placing the child over a wedge
    c. Using biofeedback
    d. Performing a visual scanning activity

84. An OT is treating a child that has difficulty with stability because of a lack of antigravity muscle strength. The BEST intervention for the OT to use is:
    a. Increasing muscle elongation
    b. Blocking or fixing certain joints
    c. Promoting equilibrium reactions
    d. Facilitating righting reactions

85. Using a medical–restorative model, the OT would provide the following intervention:
    a. Instruct a client on total hip precautions
    b. Teach compensatory techniques for loss of sensation
    c. Conduct a socialization group for several mental health patients
    d. Work on feeding and hygiene with an Alzheimer's patient

86. A patient with emphysema complains of shortness of breath and generalized weakness in the upper extremities when performing daily chores. The OT should encourage:
    a. Pursed lip breathing when working
    b. Gravity assisted exercises before performing chores
    c. Use of oxygen with daily activities
    d. Avoidance of activities that consume a lot of energy

87. When working with a patient with severe perceptual dysfunction, the therapist should:
    a. Incorporate exercise to help build strength on the involved side
    b. Focus on large components of the activity with emphasis on verbal explanation and demonstration of each component
    c. Provide as many tactile cues as possible paired as appropriate with verbal cues
    d. Utilize sidelying as much as possible to increase sensation and proprioceptive feedback on the uninvolved side

88. A spinal cord injury patient who can breathe on his own uses a sip and puff switch to operate his power wheelchair and environmental control unit and a mouthstick for writing, table games, and the computer would MOST likely have a spinal cord injury at this level:
    a. C3
    b. C4
    c. C5
    d. C6

89. The highest level of spinal cord injury at which you would expect a client to become independent in all self-care and driving with equipment would be:
    a. C7
    b. C8
    c. C5
    d. C6

90. You are treating a client that recently has a spinal cord injury at C5. The BEST piece of equipment to the client with feeding, hygiene, grooming, writing, and driving a power wheelchair would be:

a. Deltoid assist
b. Weighted pulley
c. Mobile arm supports
d. Suspension sling

91. The MOST beneficial piece of adaptive equipment to aid a client with C6 tetraplegia to work toward independence with lower extremity dressing is:
a. A trigger reacher to get the pants over the feet
b. Loops to manipulate the lower extremities
c. A universal cuff to assist with grip and closures
d. A standard dressing stick

92. With adaptive equipment and set up, the patient can perform self-feeding and engage in light hygiene, grooming, and upper extremity dressing with minimal assistance, as well as writing and use of a computer but requires an attendant to perform all other self-care. The OT would generally expect to see these goals achieved with a patient that has a spinal cord injury at level:
a. C4
b. C5
c. C6
d. C7

93. The BEST activity for someone with a visual field deficit is:
a. Reading from a book
b. Making a calendar
c. Balloon batting
d. Completing a crossword puzzle

94. The MOST appropriate model to use with clients with central nervous system dysfunction is:
a. Model of Human Occupation (MOHO)
b. Rehabilitation model
c. Biomechanical model
d. Motor control model

95. During an intervention session, the OT simulates the need for the client to walk up stairs to a kitchen with a painful/weak left leg. The patient should be instructed to move the:
a. Left leg up to the next step with the cane
b. Right leg up to the next step with the cane
c. Right leg up and then his left leg/cane
d. Left leg up and then his right leg/cane

96. OTs use all of the following modalities during intervention except:

a. Adaptive clothing
b. Work simplification and energy conservation
c. Use of physical agent modalities
d. Use of communication devices and environmental controls

97. A client with a head injury is confused and has situational disorientation and short-term memory problems. The BEST intervention to use to address the problem is:
a. Place a calendar and schedule in the client's room
b. Have the client keep a daily journal with the OT's assistance
c. Set a clock timer to remind the patient when activities are scheduled
d. Keep a checklist of the day's activities and when they are accomplished

98. A client with ideomotor apraxia would MOST likely:
a. Grasp a washcloth and be unable to sequence the movement
b. Grab the washcloth but appear unsure of how to use the soap
c. Grab the washcloth and the soap but only wash one side of the body
d. Grab the soap and the washcloth but be unable to maintain balance

99. An OT is reading the chart on a new client with a traumatic brain injury. The issue relating MOST to the client's outcome in occupational therapy would be:
a. The extent of the tissue damage
b. The amount of diffuse axonal injury
c. The presence of associated skull fractures
d. The amount of time spent in posttraumatic amnesia

100. The MOST appropriate piece of adaptive equipment for an individual with a mild to moderate left CVA would be:
a. Button hook
b. Universal cuff
c. Card holder
d. Dressing loops

101. An intervention that would benefit a client with hypotonia in the extremities and trunk is:
a. Performing fast brushing over the entire trunk and extremities
b. Slowly stretching each extremity
c. Wrapping the patient in a heavy blanket
d. Providing relaxing auditory stimulation

102. The role of an OT during a feeding group is MOST appropriate during this phase:

    a.   Oral preparatory and oral phases

    b.   Oral and pharyngeal phases

    c.   Pharyngeal and esophageal phases

    d.   Oral preparatory, oral, pharyngeal, and esophageal phases

103. The MOST common compensation principle for a client who has weakness is:

    a.   Let gravity assist

    b.   Use adaptive equipment or methods to replace lost functions, such as grasp

    c.   Use powered equipment

    d.   Use heavy utensils to increase stability

104. In general, which is the MOST appropriate ADL accommodation for hemiplegia?

    a.   Weighted items

    b.   Lightweight items

    c.   Assistive equipment

    d.   Adapted techniques

105. An OT is providing intervention for a client who had a stroke involving Broca's region in the left hemisphere. This client would have difficulty with:

    a.   Expression

    b.   Receptive language

    c.   Both expressive and receptive language

    d.   A rapid speech pattern

106. Clients demonstrating a left visual field deficit are more likely to have difficulty learning to use compensatory strategies than patients demonstrating a right visual field deficit because:

    a.   Clients read from left to right so it is easier to scan from left to right

    b.   Clients with a left hemispheric lesion usually retain scanning skills

    c.   Clients with a right hemispheric lesion usually have extensive cognitive lesions

    d.   Clients with a right hemispheric lesions always demonstrate left neglect

107. A technique frequently used for improving postural control and improving stability in the scapulohumeral area is:

    a.   Sensory integration

    b.   Weight training

    c.   Standing table

    d.   Upper extremity weight bearing

108. When a child is able to organize a successful, goal-directed action on the environment, it is referred to as a(n):
    a. Inner drive
    b. Sensory nourishment
    c. Adaptive response
    d. Sensory diet

109. An enriched environment with appropriate stimulation will cause positive brain change in the growing child. This concept may be referred to as:
    a. Just right challenge
    b. Inner drive
    c. Neural plasticity
    d. Child development

110. The child is unable to assume prone extension or maintain it when placed by the therapist. The OT would write this in which portion of the report:
    a. Subjective
    b. Clinical observations
    c. Standardized testing
    d. Functional limitations

111. Although the patient is quite thin, when the patient looks in the mirror the patient believes that they looks overweight. This patient has an inaccurate:
    a. Self-concept
    b. Body image
    c. Body scheme
    d. Seriation concept

112. A tool that helps to decrease directional confusion and facilitate a mature pencil grasp during writing activities is:
    a. A pencil grip
    b. Lined paper
    c. A smaller diameter pencil
    d. A vertical writing surface

113. A client being treated in outpatient therapy for extensor tendon repair missed three appointments while sick with the flu. When writing the monthly report, the therapist explained why the client did not achieve her short-term goals in the time frame specified. Which is the MOST appropriate section of the subjective, objective, assessment, and plan (SOAP) note for this documentation?
    a. S
    b. O
    c. A
    d. P

114. After talking to nursing, the inpatient rehab OT treated the patient in the room for instruction in safety and adaptive equipment for toileting, along with dressing and grooming activities. The patient was motivated and worked hard throughout the treatment session. Which is the BEST choice for the subjective portion of the daily SOAP note?
    a. Patient was cooperative and engaged in social conversation throughout the treatment session.
    b. Patient reports that the patient feels good today.
    c. Patient is unable to move her right upper extremity as well today as yesterday, although it doesn't really hurt but feels "tight."
    d. Nursing staff reports that patient is unsafe to toilet independently.

115. After a stroke, a patient had difficulty picking up pills from the table, difficulty buttoning, and completing jigsaw puzzles, which was a favorite leisure activity. During part of the treatment session, the patient worked on putting in and removing pieces from a jigsaw puzzle, and practice manipulating different sized coins from a flat table surface. When documenting the treatment, the BEST choice for an objective statement is:
    a. Patient worked for 15 minutes placing and removing jigsaw puzzle pieces
    b. Patient worked on tripod grasp using various coins and jigsaw puzzle pieces
    c. Patient worked for 15 minutes on tripod grasp in order to be able to grasp objects used for leisure activities and ADLs
    d. Patient worked on tripod grasp to be able to perform leisure activities and ADLs

116. Which statement would be documented in the "plan" portion of a SOAP note?
    a. Problems include decreased coordination, strength, sensation, and proprioception in left upper extremity.
    b. In order to return to work, patient will demonstrate increase of 10# of grasp in L hand, in 3 weeks.
    c. Patient would benefit from further instruction in total hip precautions for LB dressing, bathing, and hygiene.
    d. Patient attended job skills group with prompting by nursing and OT staff.

117. The parents of a child in kindergarten need instruction in the wear and care of their child's hand splint. They should also be cautioned to:
    a. Note and report to the OT any irritation and pressure problems
    b. Use disinfectants regularly to destroy bacterial growth

    c. Let the child's tolerance determine the wearing schedule

    d. Avoid putting the splint in the trunk of the car

118. An infant's parents want to watch the OT work with their child on the neonatal intensive care unit. Using a client-centered approach, the OT should:

    a. Tell the parents to leave during treatment because too many people in the room can be distracting

    b. Schedule a time to talk to the parents, different from the therapy session

    c. Ask the parents to get permission for the doctor before sharing updates on the child

    d. Offer instruction on handling and positioning

119. An elderly client using a hearing aid, eyeglasses, and a night-light is making use of:

    a. Over-the-counter remedies

    b. Assessments

    c. Props

    d. Interventions

120. The OT instructs the family of a preschooler with athetoid cerebral palsy on feeding. To maintain jaw control, the OT should recommend:

    a. Placing fingers on face to create chin tuck and manipulate mandible

    b. Vibrating the child's gums and teeth prior to feeding

    c. Holding tightly to the child's lower jaw for control

    d. Stimulating the child's upper lip by tapping to get closure

121. A patient with a kyphotic posture would possibly have difficulty putting on which type of garment?

    a. Socks

    b. Button down top

    c. Belt

    d. Pull over

122. In a skilled nursing facility, to compensate for diminished taste and sense of smell in an elderly patient, the OT should:

    a. Emphasize texture and appeal of food

    b. Recommend a diet of puree food

    c. Consult the speech therapist

    d. Emphasize eating highly seasoned food

123. The OT performs an ergonomic evaluation of an employee's computer workstation. One recommendation to the employee is to

perform stretching of the extremities and back every 30–45 minutes. What category of ergonomic intervention is this an example of?
a. Engineering control
b. Work practice control
c. Administrative control
d. Rehabilitative control

124. The OT performs an ergonomic evaluation of an employee's workstation at a manufacturing plant. The OT recommends modifying the workstation by raising the height of the assembly line by approximately 5 inches and suspending a counterbalanced power screwdriver overhead. These ergonomic interventions are considered:
a. Engineering control
b. Work practice control
c. Administrative control
d. Rehabilitative control

125. After performing ergonomic evaluations of several production lines involving 30 employees at a pharmaceutical manufacturing facility, the OT recommends a reduction in productivity rates and limited overtime and introduces job rotation for all production lines. These ergonomic interventions are considered:
a. Engineering control
b. Work practice control
c. Administrative control
d. Rehabilitative control

126. The MOST effective OT intervention recommendation to prevent a client from developing a work-related wrist and hand musculoskeletal disorder is:
a. Personal protective equipment such as padded work gloves
b. Work practice controls such as stretching
c. Engineering controls such as workstation modification
d. Administrative controls such as job rotation

127. The OT is trying to facilitate the appropriate finger grasp pattern of a child around 8–9 months of age by having the child trap a small cracker between the thumb IP joint and radial side of his flexed index finger. The therapist is working to facilitate the:
a. Three-jaw chuck
b. Inferior pincer grasp
c. Radial digital grasp
d. Raking grasp

128. A child in occupational therapy is throwing a tennis ball at a target. It is likely that the OT is trying to develop a:
    a. Radial digital grasp
    b. Cylindrical grasp
    c. Disc grasp
    d. Spherical grasp

129. An OT is assisting a child with positioning scissors. The OT wants to be sure that the child is using the scissors appropriately. It is likely that the OT will cue the child to hold the scissors by:
    a. Placing the child's thumb in one loop and four remaining fingers in the other loop of the scissors
    b. Placing the child's thumb and index finger in the loops of the scissors, with the middle finger resting against the shaft of the handle
    c. Placing the child's thumb and middle finger in the loops of the scissors, with the index finger resting against the shaft of the handle
    d. Telling the child to the hold the scissors "like a big boy"

130. An OT presents a child with 10 pictures and asks the child to pick out 2 that are the same. It is MOST likely that the OT is facilitating the child's development of:
    a. Visual discrimination abilities
    b. Spatial perception abilities
    c. Visual closure abilities
    d. Visual pursuit abilities

131. The OT is consulting with a speech and language pathologist on positioning of a child who has cerebral palsy with increased tone. The speech and language pathologist wants the child to observe her mouth and repeat what the speech and language pathologist says. It is likely that the OT will recommend that the child be seated in the child's wheelchair with the speech and language pathologist:
    a. Standing above the child so that the child looks up
    b. Standing behind the child so that the child turns around
    c. Sitting beside the child so that the child turns to her side
    d. Sitting directly in front of the child so that the child looks forward

132. The OT is providing services to a child with spastic hemiplegia. The child demonstrates an associated grasp on the affected side when using the unaffected hand, thus making difficult for the child to engage in bilateral tasks. The child would like to take off their shoes. It is likely that the OT will suggest that the child:
    a. Sit on a chair with a high back and hold on to the chair with one hand while using a dressing hook to push off the shoes one at a time

b. Sit on a low stool so that both of his feet are on the floor while holding onto the stool with both hands for support and pushing the child's shoes off one at time by digging the child's heel into the ground

c. Lay supine on the child's bed and flex the child's hips and knees so that the child can reach his feet to pull off the shoes one at a time

d. Sit on a chair and cross one leg over the other so that the child can reach down and remove each shoe one at a time

133. The OT is consulting with a special education preschool teacher who leads a class of children with significant motor involvement. The teacher describes one student who has an open-mouthed posture and drools throughout the day. The teacher would like to assist this student in maintaining a closed mouth and swallowing his saliva periodically. It is likely that the OT will recommend that the teacher:

a. Support the child by placing her middle finger just behind the chin, with the index finger and thumb wrapping around either side of the child's jaw

b. Provide the child with a bib or washcloth to absorb the drool and prevent any from getting on the child's clothing

c. Place the index finger in a horizontal position between the child's upper lip and nose and provide firm and continuous pressure

d. Remind the student to close the student's mouth and swallow while modeling this behavior

134. The OT is working with a child on reaching for toys. In order to prepare the child for reaching, the OT first facilitates dynamic weight bearing and weight shifting on elbows and hands. The OT intervention is MOST likely guided by the principles of:

a. Biomechanical model

b. NDT

c. Sensory Integration theory

d. MOHO

135. The OT is treating an 18-month-old child with significant motor impairments. The OT would like to introduce the child to assistive technology so that the child may produce greater effects within the context of his home. The OT might first introduce him to a(n):

a. Augmentative communication device

b. Environmental controls

c. Single switch

d. Computer with touch screen

136. An infant in the neonatal intensive care unit is being transitioned from a nasogastric tube to a bottle for feeding. When presented with the bottle, the infant demonstrates aversive responses, such as arching away, crying, and grimacing. The OT is working to minimize the child's aversive response to oral-tactile stimuli. It is likely that to address this concern that the OT will:
    a. Modify the characteristics of the infant's food
    b. Provide graded tactile input
    c. Position the child in a position to support physiologic function
    d. Recommend supplemental feedings

137. The OT is working with a 5-year-old child to develop pre-writing skills. The child has adequate fine motor strength, eye-hand coordination, ability to hold a writing utensil, and the capacity to make circles and letters. However, the child is unable to perceive the differences between letters. During a treatment session, the OT will likely encourage the child to:
    a. Play a matching game
    b. Pick up small items with tweezers
    c. Complete dot-to-dot pictures and mazes
    d. Maneuver through an obstacle course

138. The OT is working with a group of first-grade students. As the children copy a four-word sentence, the OT observes that the children are having difficulty leaving large enough spaces in between words. The OT might encourage the children to:
    a. Skip lines on the paper
    b. Use paper with raised writing lines as tactile cues for letter placement
    c. Use grid paper
    d. Place a penny at the end of one word before writing the next one

139. A 4-year-old child presents with significant motor delays. The focus of occupational therapy is to assist the child in grasping toys. MOST likely, the OT will first address:
    a. Voluntary hand opening
    b. Carrying the object
    c. Supination
    d. Finger flexion

140. An 8-year-old child is receiving occupational therapy to address functional bilateral hand skills. The child has a great deal of difficulty with refined movements. Before presenting the child with greater challenges, the OT will first engage the child in:

a. Performing a two-dimensional art project
b. Playing catch with a large inflatable beach ball
c. Cutting out complex shapes
d. Playing a video game with a handheld controller

141. The OT has provided a fourth-grade student with a built-up pencil grip, but the student continues to hold his pencil too tightly and presses very hard on the paper when writing. At times the student presses so hard that the paper tears. MOST likely the OT will provide this student with:
    a. A notebook to write on top of
    b. A tape recorder to dictate the work
    c. Worksheets to practice handwriting
    d. A thicker pencil

142. A school-based OT is working with a student who has an autism spectrum disorder. The child engages in sensory seeking behavior by crashing into the lockers while walking in the hallway. In order to support the student in adaptively responding to the environment before entering the hallway, the OT will likely provide the student with:
    a. Vestibular input in the form of swinging on a doorway swing in the classroom
    b. Proprioceptive input in the form of joint compression applied to upper and lower extremities
    c. Tactile input in the form of finger painting
    d. Visual input in the form of a picture that explains where they are going in the school building

143. A 3-year-old child with a diagnosis of developmental coordination disorder is being seen in a private clinic for occupational therapy. The OT sets up an obstacle course and encourages the child to explore it. It is MOST likely that the OT is trying to:
    a. Support the child's development of automatic motor responses in novel situations
    b. Assess whether or not the child demonstrates an aversive response to having both feet off the ground
    c. Provide the child with opportunities to increase trunk and upper extremity strength
    d. Help the child develop essential pre-academic skills

144. A preterm infant has difficulty maintaining lip seal on a bottle's nipple during feeding. The OT can support this child's participation in feeding by:
    a. Touching the child's cheek to elicit the rooting reflex

b. Swaddling the baby with arms and legs tucked in towards the midline or with hands by face

c. Positioning the infant in an upright sidelying position to simulate the position of breast feeding

d. Providing firm, steady jaw support externally under the base of the tongue and firm, but gentle cheek support

145. You are working with a 45-year-old patient who is recovering from a C5 spinal cord injury. The patient is tetraplegic and you are addressing self-feeding during your treatment session. During your session the patient's legs began to bounce up and down repeatedly to the extent that the patient's arms are shaking from the movement and the patient is unable to continue to self-feed. Your BEST course of action would be the following:

a. Make the room warmer as this will make the patient's legs stop shaking

b. Use a Hoyer lift to transfer the patient onto a bed or mat to stop the shaking

c. Ask the patient to stop feeding and relax so the shaking will stop

d. Provide weight bearing through the patient's knees toward the patient's ankles to stop the shaking

146. An 18-year-old patient who sustained a severe brain injury 6 months ago is seeing you for therapy. The patient's finger flexion spasticity is now to the point of being painful with passive movement of fingers to 0 degrees and 20 degrees of wrist flexion. Pain also begins with 20-degree wrist extension if the fingers are flexed. The thumb is adducted into the palm. Which splint would be BEST for this patient?

a. A dorsal-based forearm splint with finger separators

b. Neoprene thumb abduction splint

c. A volar-based forearm splint with cone shaped hand piece

d. A soft prefabricated hand splint

147. You currently work in an outpatient clinic and have evaluated a 35-year-old patient who is status post–3 months from a spinal cord injury at the level of C6. The patient's upper extremity function is consistent with his stated level of injury. Which of the long-term goals is unrealistic?

a. Patient will be independent with bathing utilizing adaptive equipment

b. Patient will be independent with eating precut food after set-up and adaptive equipment as needed

c. Patient will dress upper body independently after set-up

d. Patient will be independent with directing bowel and bladder care

148. As a home health therapist, you are treating a 55-year-old who has a very supportive spouse and a caregiver during the day who helps

with self-care and other tasks needed in the home. The patient enjoys their children and grandchildren who live in the immediate area. The patient is currently in stage 3 of amyotrophic lateral sclerosis, with severe weakness of the ankles, wrists, and hands. The patient minimally ambulates and fatigues easily. An appropriate intervention would be:

a. Light strengthening program
b. Help prioritize activities and provide work simplification
c. Learning how to cook three-course meals
d. Worksite assessment

149. You are working with an 18-year-old who has a C5 spinal cord injury. The patient has not begun to self-feed. Based on the level of the injury, a piece of equipment that would benefit the client is:

a. Wrist splint with u-cuff
b. u-cuff
c. No equipment needed
d. Tenodesis splint

150. You are working with a 47-year-old client who has a spinal cord injury. The client demonstrates some hypertonicty in the upper extremities. A method to perform ROM while preserving tenodisis is:

a. Wrist flexed, fingers extended
b. Wrist extended, fingers extended
c. Wrist radial deviated, fingers extended
d. Functional position

151. You are currently seeing a 16-year-old who has sustained a traumatic brain injury and is in the hospital waiting to transfer to a rehabilitation center. The client is beginning to exhibit hypertonus and tight fisting of both hands. You decide to fabricate bilateral hand splints for the following goal:

a. Prevent skin breakdown
b. Prevent contracture
c. Increase functional use
d. a and b

152. Using an adaptive approach, one way to suggest for someone to modify the home for decreased acuity would be to:

a. Use non-slip rugs
b. Increase light while minimizing glare
c. Notify neighbors of the problem
d. Encourage driving cessation

153. You are working with a 70-year-old patient who sustained a left parietal stroke 10 months ago, and the family reports that they want the patient to see on the right side. The patient has just

completed outpatient therapy at a nearby facility. You decide to use an adaptive approach and family education with this patient. An example of the strategies you may suggest include:
a. Providing computer retraining so that the patient will learn to look to the right side
b. Placing all necessary items on the right side of the patient
c. Providing scanning worksheets that are placed in midline and cue the patient to make sure the patient looks to the right when completing the activity
d. Placing the TV remote control consistently on the patient's right side

154. You are working in the hospital and receive a consult to see a 65-year-old patient who has recently had a left CVA. When you enter the room and explain the role and purpose of occupational therapy, the patient immediately states the desire to brush the patient's hair. As the patient reaches for the brush and then brushes their hair with their right hand, you notice that although the patient has adequate ROM, to complete the task the patient has difficulty with the fine adjustments needed to brush the patient's hair. You then know that the following deficit area requires further evaluation:
a. Attention
b. Sequencing
c. Spatial neglect
d. Motor apraxia

155. While an OT is working with a patient during an ADL session, the patient begins to dress the OT's arms instead of the patient's arms. This can be BEST described as:
a. Somatagnosia
b. Difficulty with sequencing
c. Spatial neglect
d. None of the above

156. You are treating a 20-year-old patient who sustained a brain injury 10 months ago. The patient recently moved into a group home and is learning to regain independence. In therapy, the patient recently achieved the goal of doing laundry independently. When the patient returned to therapy, the patient reported that the patient was unable to complete her laundry at the group home. This would be called difficulty with:
a. Social skills
b. Generalization
c. Sequencing
d. Attention

157. You have been referred a 32-year-old parent of two young children who has been recently diagnosed for multiple sclerosis. Your evaluation reveals that the patient's performance skills of motor control and cognition are all within normal limits. Education of the patient should include:
    a.   End of life issues
    b.   Energy conservation
    c.   Memory strategies
    d.   Bathroom modification ideas

158. You are treating a C7 spinal cord injury patient who is working on independent feeding. One way to grade this activity would be to:
    a.   Provide built-up handle utensils
    b.   Provide plate guard
    c.   Go from eating pudding to steak
    d.   Provide a u-cuff

159. You are working with a 35-year-old client who has sustained a right CVA and demonstrates a left inattention. Your remedial strategies might include:
    a.   Providing tactile cues to the left side
    b.   Placing the television on the right side of the room
    c.   Placing all of the client's items on the right side of the client's body
    d.   All of the above

160. You are working with a 53-year-old client who has had a right CVA. The patient is lying on a therapy mat and you are performing passive ROM to her left arm. Once you have the patient's arm in 90 degrees of flexion, the patient complains of some discomfort and pain. The BEST course of action would be:
    a.   Continue as tolerated, because passive ROM must be maintained
    b.   Begin the ROM again and make sure the scapula is gliding
    c.   Continue and do not go past the point of pain
    d.   Consult an orthopedic specialist

161. A patient with a C5 spinal cord injury has been admitted to the inpatient rehab unit for therapy. To teach self-feeding, the OT might use adaptive equipment such as:
    a.   Built-up handle utensils
    b.   A mobile arm support
    c.   Dynamic tenodesis splints
    d.   Short opponens splints

162. A patient admitted to the geriatric unit with a diagnosis of Alzheimer's disease can no longer live alone. A family member is now planning to have the patient move into the family member's home. The primary focus of the OT intervention will MOST likely consist of:
    a. Maximizing the patient's current cognitive perceptual skills
    b. Improving the patient's level of independence with ADL tasks
    c. Training the patient and family in the use of adaptive and bathroom equipment
    d. Providing caregiver training with strategies on how to adapt tasks or the environment

163. An 11-month-old continues to have formula as a primary source of nutrition. There are oral structural changes that occur as the child nears 12 months of age, and feeding in a reclined position would increase the possibility of aspiration. Which of the following oral structural changes make it imperative for the child to feed in an upright sitting position?
    a. The epiglottis and soft palate are in direct proximation
    b. The hyoid, larynx, and epiglottis ascend
    c. The oral cavity is small with fatty cheeks and the tongue
    d. The pharynx is elongated

164. A 12-month-old with oral hypersensitivity and extreme aversion to textured food. The child spits, gags, or coughs whenever pureed food is offered. This is a critical problem, because it limits nutritional intake. The BEST intervention activity would be:
    a. Use salty and sweet foods alternatively on the tongue
    b. Apply vibration to the mouth and near the vestibular receptors
    c. Consult with a nutritionist regarding the effect of dietary change
    d. Place food on the posterior part of the tongue for improved tolerance

165. A 7-year-old with athetoid cerebral palsy exhibits poor arm and hand control. A strategy that would help with self-feeding is:
    a. Using a spoon with a built-up handle
    b. Placing in a high chair
    c. Using a wider and flatter dish
    d. Providing foot support

166. A 1-year-old infant with autism has oral hypersensitivity. The BEST intervention to help the child cope would be:
    a. Soft white bread
    b. Dried fruits and pretzels
    c. Soft crackers and cookies
    d. Raw vegetables

167. A 12-month-old has respiratory problems and sometimes requires oxygen support. Rapid and shallow breathing hamper the child's ability to swallow because it interferes with the coordination of the suck-swallow-breathe sequence. This would be remedied if the child's breathing were slowed down. A strategy that would benefit the child during intervention is:
    a. Place the child in an upright position while feeding
    b. Use thickened liquid for greater proprioceptive input
    c. Use a neck flexion and improve closure of the larynx
    d. Use oral vibration

168. An 8-year-old exhibits hyperextension of the trunk and neck and has a tonic bite. A strategy that would promote improved oral motor control during feeding would be:
    a. Seating him in a beanbag chair for feeding
    b. Using a spoon to create downward pressure on the center of his tongue
    c. Using a bolster under his arms for support
    d. Applying touch pressure on his cheeks

169. A 16-month-old and has significant motor problems. Drinking is a more difficult skill for the child to achieve than eating solid foods. An appropriate liquid to include in the child's daily feedings would be:
    a. Encourage the child to have vegetable broth
    b. Make sure the child drinks water
    c. Include thick cream soups in the diet
    d. Provide fruit juices with a thin consistency

170. A 5-year-old child with neuromuscular dystrophy is undergoing occupational therapy. While dressing the child is extremely impatient and gets discouraged when not able to dress correctly. An intervention approach that could be used is:
    a. Restore approach
    b. Backward chaining
    c. Forward chaining
    d. Adaptatory approach

171. A 4-year-old has moderate motor limitations. An OT is helping the child with brushing teeth and bathing. A tool that would be helpful in this process is:
    a. Trunk support
    b. Weighted tooth brush
    c. Enlarged tooth brush handle
    d. Electric toothbrush

172. A 7-year-old child displays limited writing performance in class and often rests its head on the desktop while writing. Sometimes,

the child slips out of his chair. The OT decides that the child would benefit from a handwriting intervention program with preparatory activities, such as calisthenics. This would include pushups on the floor, resistive exercises with the Thera-Band, and writing in the prone position. Selection of this type of preparatory intervention would be because:

a. Muscle tone needs to be decreased
b. Energy levels need to be increased
c. Proximal strength and stability need to be improved
d. Proprioceptive feedback needs to be enhanced

173. A child exhibits muscle tension when holding a pencil by exerting too much pressure while writing and often tears the paper. The OT wants to modify the grip pattern. A remedial intervention that could be used is:
    a. Teach him to use a mature grasp
    b. Give him an unconventional writing tool
    c. Introduce a rubber-band sling
    d. Teach him to use wider-lined paper

174. A preparatory activity for handwriting is to listen to rhythmic music while sitting in a rocking chair. The model of practice that this relates to is:
    a. Sensorimotor
    b. Psychosocial
    c. Biomechanical
    d. Psychoeducational

175. A child has difficulty in placing cursive letters on the line and spacing words and does not use margins properly. Sixty percent of the child's work is not legible. The child gets poor grades not because of lack of content but because of lack of legibility. A compensatory intervention that would help is:
    a. Give more oral assignments
    b. Allow use of a computer for all schoolwork
    c. Use smaller-lined paper and write on every line
    d. Use fingerprint spacing using an ink pad before finger spacing

176. A 6-year-old has managed to write some of the easier manuscript letters, such as o, l, and t, but has difficulty in writing letters such as b, q, and g. An intervention strategy to use with this child would be:
    a. Introduce letters with common formational features as one group
    b. Reinforce newly acquired letters by getting him to write them repeatedly

    c. Have him write the letters repeatedly on a blackboard while standing

    d. Choose a commercially available handwriting intervention method and follow it strictly

177. An OT may have to direct and guide functional written communication by using a combination of compensatory and remedial intervention approaches. A remedial handwriting intervention plan for handwriting would be:

    a. Include more oral activities

    b. Add cushions and a foot rest to the student's desk

    c. Use adhesive strips as spacers between words

    d. Move the student's desk away from the window to the middle of the room

178. A second grader has illegible script, and the OT feels that along with remedial techniques the child would benefit from compensatory activities using the sensorimotor approach. The OT recommends use of chalk or grease pencils as writing tools to improve legibility. The reasoning behind this is:

    a. It will provide additional proprioceptive input

    b. It will provide a structured manner for writing

    c. It will provide strength to the hand

    d. It can alleviate fatigue

179. A fourth-grade student has difficulty holding down more than one key on a keyboard simultaneously and uses only one hand at a time. A possible intervention strategy that the OT could suggest is:

    a. Change the height of table or chair

    b. Use an expanded keyboard with larger keys

    c. Use a chord keyboard

    d. Add cushioning around the keyboard

180. A 7-year-old with motor limitations gets tired doing writing assignments and has poor handwriting. The OT feels that making a transition from handwriting to text generation would help the child. A software program that would help the child is:

    a. Imagination Letter series

    b. Abbreviation expansion

    c. Talking word processor

    d. Early Learning House Series

181. A 3-year-old has spina bifida and needs mobility augmentation to be able to move outdoors, in hallways, and in corridors. A mobility device that could be recommended would be:

    a. Hand-propelled tricycle model

    b. Supine scooter

    c. Aeroplane mobility device

    d. Crocodile posterior walker

182. An 18-month-old with arthrogryposis is alert, sensitive, and very eager to explore the environment. The therapy team wants to use a mobility device that allows the child to be in an upright, hands-free, weight-bearing position, while providing active ROM. Because the child will be moving about inside a small apartment, an important requirement is that the device allows for a high degree of maneuverability. A mobility device that would be MOST suitable for this child would be:

    a. The aeroplane mobility device

    b. The Transitional Ortho-Therapeutic Walker (TOTWalker)

    c. The ABLER, a mobile stander

    d. Crocodile posterior walker

183. A 5-year-old with moderate spastic diplegia uses a push walker, but the OT has recommended a manual wheelchair for mobility in the school and community. A feature that would allow for independent transfer in and out of the chair would be:

    a. Large front tires

    b. Wheel locks

    c. Higher seat height

    d. Increased height of push handles

184. A preterm infant born at 34 weeks' gestation. The infant had transient respiratory distress of the newborn (TRDN) for which oxygen was given from an oxyhood for 48 hours. Oral feedings began on the third day and intake was fairly good. The physician had ordered a transition from a regular 3-hour feeding schedule to cue-based oral feeding for the infant. The nurse has observed that the infant feeds well initially and then becomes disorganized and tachypneic. An approach that would ensure the infant feeds without compromising nutrition would be:

    a. To receive nasogastric tube (NGT) feedings only

    b. To be fed a preset volume for a preset duration of time

    c. To feed only till cues suggest stress and fatigue

    d. To feed by a percutaneous endoscopic gastrostomy tube

185. Therapy occurs at home for a child who exhibits developmental delays because of Down syndrome. In this natural learning environment, various activities and learning experiences occur. An activity that the child could participate in which would be a structured would be:

    a. Playing at the playground

    b. Attending a mother–infant playgroup

    c. Hippotherapy

    d. Regularly playing in the sandbox

186. A 6-year-old receives occupational therapy for improving fine motor functions. An activity that would help improve eye-hand coordination is:
    a. Playing with toy hammer and nails
    b. Practicing in-hand manipulation by rotating small objects in her hand
    c. Rolling Play Doh into a ball
    d. Finger painting using shaving cream

187. An 8-year-old has had a spinal cord injury and is in acute care. Assessment would also include evaluation of the need for specialized equipment. What specialized equipment would be necessary for use in the hospital and after discharge?
    a. Pressure garment
    b. Splints
    c. Adapted toilet seat
    d. Adapted utensils

188. A bulimic patient that you are working with is in a day treatment program. Which of the following activities would you MOST likely use with the patient during treatment?
    a. Simple craft kits
    b. Time management groups
    c. Stress management groups
    d. Reminiscence groups

189. A bipolar I patient with manic symptoms has been on your unit many times. You know that this patient is fond of you, but this time shocks you by greeting you with a confession of love and a marriage proposal. Which of the following would be your BEST response?
    a. Tell the patient that it is a ridiculous thing to say and you'll have the nurse prescribe more medication
    b. Tell the patient that, of course, you are flattered, but that your role is to work together in occupational therapy and it is extremely important that you maintain a professional relationship in order to provide the best quality of care
    c. Let the patient know that you do think that the patient is "kind of cute" and maybe something can be worked out after they leave the hospital
    d. Tell the patient that it is inappropriate behavior, which must stop immediately

190. The BEST occupational therapy intervention for a patient with a generalized anxiety disorder would be:
    a. 1000-piece puzzle
    b. Relay races

    c. Assertiveness training

    d. Deep-breathing and relaxation exercises

191. A well-respected professor recently suffered the loss of a spouse and only child in an automobile accident. The client feels guilty for not being in the car with them and was unable to prevent the tragedy. The client is obviously suffering from depression and has now lost all interest and motivation in normal daily activities and has stopped habitual performance of a balanced lifestyle. The client feels that the client has no control over the client's "world" and what happens any more. The client knows that their suicidal thoughts are not healthy, but the client says that they lack the skills to make things better. The BEST framework to use in your approach to evaluating this client is:
    a. MOHO
    b. Developmental Frame of Reference
    c. Cognitive Disabilities Frame of Reference
    d. Behavioral Frame of Reference

192. Which occupational therapy frame of reference or model of practice, used in mental health intervention, emphasizes that assessment is the MOST important role for the OT?
    a. MOHO
    b. Developmental Frame of Reference
    c. Cognitive Disabilities Frame of Reference
    d. Person-Environment-Occupation Performance Model (PEO)

193. Which of the following statements is true for the Cognitive Disabilities Frame of Reference?
    a. Patients can learn new skills to improve their performance of tasks
    b. Making environmental changes can enhance a client's performance
    c. A person's measured cognitive level can fluctuate greatly
    d. It is only useful with the chronically mentally ill

194. When applying a Psychoanalytic Frame of Reference perspective to mental health occupational therapy intervention:
    a. Psychopathology is believed to be the result of faulty learning.
    b. Occupation can be used to uncover unconscious drives and feelings.
    c. Cognitive functioning is the result of a physical or chemical dysfunction in the brain.
    d. The environment must be adapted to positively impact the patient's functioning.

195. Directive group formats used under MOHO will:
    a. Vary in routine and organization
    b. Provide practice in advanced communication and assertiveness techniques
    c. Use co-leadership whenever possible
    d. Expect patients to be able to tolerate a minimum of 1-hour sessions for skill development

196. Systematic desensitization and exposure techniques used with phobic patients stem from which framework?
    a. Developmental Frame of Reference
    b. Behavioral Frame of Reference
    c. MOHO
    d. Psychoanalytical Frame of Reference

197. In an effort to shape the behavior of your patient during treatment you choose to reinforce a certain behavior every single time that it is demonstrated. What schedule of reinforcement does this represent?
    a. Continuous
    b. Intermittent
    c. Fixed ratio
    d. Fixed interval

198. You are treating an adult patient in your clinic using a psychoanalytical approach. The activity that would be MOST useful to you is:
    a. A leather cigarette case kit
    b. Pottery clay
    c. A Monopoly game
    d. A precut wooden key rack

199. The BEST treatment for children with autism involves:
    a. Sensory-motor intervention and therapy to learn self-management skills
    b. ROM and muscle strengthening
    c. Perceptual-motor training
    d. Cognitive-perceptual training

200. An occupational therapy client is experiencing extensive occupational dysfunction caused by HIV and depression. The patient reports a loss of interest in most activities, including self-care and leisure, and has a limited tolerance for any physical activity. You suspect that this is partially because of decreased self-worth and fear of failure. The BEST activities to use in initial treatment interventions might include which of the following?
    a. Leading group exercises each morning on the unit
    b. ADL practice and expressive arts

    c. Communications groups

    d. Assertiveness training

201. Using a life span developmental approach in working with older clients, a therapist might use which of the following programming in treatment?

    a. Expressive arts group

    b. Exercise group

    c. Reminiscence group

    d. Communication group

202. A 73-year-old is experiencing cognitive deficits and has limited physical capabilities because of Parkinson's disease. Which of the following would be the MOST appropriately used intervention for this client?

    a. Craft groups involving the construction a memory book

    b. Leisure planning groups to develop a plan for regular leisure involvement

    c. Exercise groups to build endurance

    d. Problem-solving groups to help him deal with life changes

203. You are leading a group on an inpatient acute care unit and your patients are mostly young schizophrenics. Attention to tasks is short and they need constant redirection to participate effectively. Which kind of group would MOST appropriately meet their needs?

    a. Psychoeducational

    b. Current events with a directive format

    c. Self-esteem building

    d. Leather crafts

204. Which of the following groups is appropriate to use for Level 2 clients when using a Cognitive Disabilities Frame of Reference?

    a. Cooking

    b. Work evaluation

    c. Grooming

    d. Movement

205. You are visiting the home of a client recently diagnosed with Alzheimer's. The environment is terribly cluttered and seems to add to the patient's current level of confusion. You decide to:

    a. Clean up the place by yourself, throw away a lot, and put everything else away properly to help organized the environment for the client

    b. Leave it alone and just recognize that this is how the person will be living

c. Engage family members in helping the client to sort through some of the cluttered items and make some choices about what to and what not to keep

d. Encourage the family to hire a housekeeper, who will make sure that the environment is clean and tidy all the time

206. You have a 17-year-old in your group who begins to act out and verbally threaten others. You've given the patient several warnings to discontinue this behavior and they have been ignored. The BEST thing to do next would be:
    a. Call security and have the client physically removed from the group
    b. Ask the client to leave the group and tell the client that if the client complies you will meet with the client later to discuss the situation
    c. Demand that the client discontinue the client's behavior and threaten the client with removal
    d. Take all the other patients out of the room and then confront the client alone

207. Which of the following activities would be MOST appropriate to use in intervention for a child with ADHD?
    a. Gross motor group
    b. Handwriting practice
    c. Social skills group
    d. Leisure skills group

208. All of the following are essential services of a Psychosocial Rehabilitation program except:
    a. Medication management
    b. Daily living skills training
    c. Vocational rehabilitation
    d. Case management

209. Which scenario represents the MOST appropriate means for OTs to use physical agents' modalities?
    a. The OT applies a hot pack to decrease stiffness of the neck and shoulder.
    b. A patient with osteoarthritis is prescribed fluidotherapy for 20 minutes to the affected extremity.
    c. Patient receives contrast heat and cryotherapy treatments to minimize edema.
    d. A patient is prescribed fluidotherapy for 20 minutes, then works on buttoning shirt.

210. The BEST example of a statement that would document the patient's prognosis is:

a. The patient may require prolonged time to perform transfers because of poor motor planning ability.
b. The patient received a home program on energy conservation and work simplification.
c. Compared to the norm, grip strength is within normal limits and age appropriate.
d. The patient performed a stand pivot transfer to and from the wheelchair to bathtub.

211. The OT is providing intervention for a patient with a right radial nerve compression. The MOST immediate action to take is to:
a. Teach alternative methods for self-feeding
b. Provide a dynamic splint for wrist drop
c. Teach ROM to prevent muscle tightness
d. Provide a forearm sling to prevent wrist drop

212. During a session on bed positioning, the OT should instruct a patient with thoracic outlet syndrome to sleep in:
a. Sidelying on the unaffected side with a pillow under the cervical region
b. A facelying position with the arms above the head
c. Sidelying on the affected side to provide proprioceptive input to the shoulder
d. Supine position with the arms above the head

213. When discharging a patient with Alzheimer's to a skilled nursing facility, what is the MOST important information to share?
a. Summary on cognitive performance
b. Recommendations to a support group
c. Summary of the patient progress
d. Results of the initial evaluation

214. Which patient should the OT recommend to use a sliding board?
a. An elderly patient with a history of falls
b. A patient wearing a leg cast
c. A patient with lower extremity weakness
d. A patient who fatigues easily

215. An OT is working with a client who exhibits deficits with upper extremity coordination. During a cooking activity, the OT might recommend that the individual:
a. Use lightweight utensils, pots, and pans
b. Place items within easy reach for greater control
c. Use one extremity at a time
d. Use heavy-weighted utensils, pots, and pans

216. The OT is providing rehab to a person who is paraplegic. When performing activities to the lower extremity, the OT should instruct the person to:
    a. Support the trunk with one extremity while performing tasks with the other
    b. Use bilateral coordination to perform lower extremity activities
    c. Perform all activities close to the midline of the body for success
    d. Secure the assistance of the caregiver

217. The OT needs to perform a dependent transfer with a person who is too weak to move independently. The BEST technique is to:
    a. Stand in front of the person and encourage standing upright, then pivoting to the side
    b. Use one person technique by standing in front of the person and placing them in a forward flexed position
    c. Ask another OT to assist; both will secure the patient under the arms and will pull into a standing position
    d. Secure a transfer belt around the individual and pull to stand

218. A patient with chronic back pain is also a mechanic and needs to be able to perform the job as it provides the only household income. What is the MOST important compensatory strategy the OT should include when advising about occupational performance?
    a. When in pain, sit to perform major tasks
    b. Reinforce body mechanics and pacing of work
    c. Work during the periods when pain has subsided
    d. Use adaptive equipment to minimize stress to joints

219. During a home health visit, a patient experiencing cancer fatigue states that the goal is to be able to prepare simple meals. What strategy should the OT suggest as the MOST efficient way to engage in this occupation?
    a. Have patient prepare the item and elicit help from caregiver for actual cooking
    b. Prepare meals on an alternating schedule about three to four times per week
    c. Organize work areas and store frequently used items in easily accessible areas
    b. Think ahead and schedule rest breaks during meal preparation and cooking

220. A client with mild dementia lives in an assisted living facility. The OT is consulted to recommend strategies to help the person maintain functional independence as long as possible. One strategy for promoting independence in occupational performance is to:

a. Have patient keep a journal of the most frequent activities during the day
b. Improve lighting in all rooms for better localization of items that will be needed daily
c. Require a buddy system in which a neighbor can remind the person of what is needed to do
d. Place picture, schedules, and items related to daily activities throughout the house

221. A patient in a wheelchair exhibits moderate postural instability and weakness in the trunk and shoulders but has fair to good hand skills. To encourage bilateral upper extremity use the OT should:
a. Place lateral supports in the wheelchair
b. Attach a lapboard to the wheelchair
c. Use a head harness to hold patient upright
d. Recline the back of the wheelchair

222. A patient with intention tremors is having difficulty with grooming activities. To promote functional performance, the OT should incorporate:
a. Using long handles on equipment used for grooming
b. Using weighted cuffs on wrists while performing grooming tasks
c. Sitting at a table to perform the grooming tasks
d. Having patient take medication prior to engaging in the activity

223. The OT is working on balancing a checkbook with a patient that has a traumatic brain injury. When the patient becomes visibly agitated, the OT should:
a. Change the activity to redirect attention
b. Stop treatment and refer to the physician
c. Suggest that medication be given
d. Wait a little while and then try again

224. The BEST strategy to use with a contracted joint that has a soft end field is to:
a. Perform tendon gliding exercises
b. Apply low load long duration stretch
c. Use a quick stretch technique
d. Perform active ROM

225. A patient complains of increased pain after receiving passive joint mobility exercise in therapy two days earlier. On examination, the OT notices redness and inflamed joints. The NEXT course of action is to:
a. Discontinue therapy
b. Use a more gentle technique for passive mobilization
c. Change to gentle active and active assist activities
d. Immobilize the affected body parts

226. Anxiety over shortness of breath may be reduced in cardiac and chronic obstructive pulmonary disorder patients by employing the stress management technique of visualization. This technique is effective because it:
    a. Helps persons to mentally transport out of the situation
    b. Promotes scanning of the environment surrounding the individual
    c. Allows person to distinguish between figure-ground concepts
    d. Allows the person to examine future goals

227. A patient in a skilled nursing facility exhibits hyposensitivity of oral motor musculature. To benefit the patient, the OT should introduce:
    a. A pureed diet
    b. Eating crunchy vegetables
    c. The use of bolus or flavorful foods
    d. A bland diet

228. The OT is consulting with an employer about the high incidences of cumulative trauma disorders in the workplace and has been asked to make recommendations about prevention. According to the OT the BEST solution for prevention of cumulative trauma is to:
    a. Assess work areas for the appropriateness of furnishing and accessories
    b. Purchase a supply of braces and Ace bandages to use for support when working
    c. Start a job rotation plan immediately
    d. Introduce employees to scheduled breaks and relaxation techniques

229. Which activities should the OT incorporate as interventions for a client with visual acuity problems?
    a. Racking horizontally and vertically
    b. Contrasting of bright, bold colors with a background
    c. Verbal cues to attend to the neglected side
    d. Tracing letter and number with the tips of the fingers

230. According to biomechanical principles, muscles too weak to resist gravity should be:
    a. Placed in a functional position
    b. Placed in an antideformity or safe position
    c. Supported by using a sling or lapboard for support
    d. Strengthened with the use of isokinetic exercise

231. Which of the following approaches might the OT use for sensory reeducation of a person following a peripheral nerve injury?
    a. Applying pressure and performing massage
    b. Object recognition, manipulation, and localization

    c. Alternately using heat and cold

    d. Using vision as compensation for deficits

232. The OT needs to employ a compensatory treatment for an individual who has sensory problems. Which strategy would be the MOST effective?

    a. Use the uninvolved extremity to test temperatures and items for safety before engaging in the activity

    b. Perform a graded program that includes applying different textures and media to a hypersensitive body part

    c. Bombard as many senses as possible to promote sensory reintegration and sensory return

    d. Perform a program to help a patient correctly interpret and differentiate between sensory stimuli

233. Which technique reflects a desensitization treatment for an individual with a sensory issue?

    a. Teaching a spinal cord injured client how to inspect the parts of the body that lack sensation

    b. Using the less affected hand to perform activities such as cooking, eating, or ironing

    c. Performing a graded therapy program that includes applying different textures and media to a sensitive part of the body

    d. Encouraging the use of vision and other senses to prevent injury specific parts of the body

234. According to occupational therapy principles, which scenario demonstrates the MOST appropriate use of therapeutic exercise?

    a. The patient performs stretching and ROM of the upper extremities, followed by a self-feeding activity.

    b. The patient performs 10 repetitions of elbow curls on the first visit and increase to 20 reps on the next visit.

    c. The patient engages in a meal preparation and cooking activity from a wheelchair.

    d. The patient performs graded isometric, isotonic, and eccentric strengthening on the same day.

235. An OT is training a patient in the principles of joint protection techniques before they are discharged. Education would focus on:

    a. Massaging a joint before exercise

    b. Using the strongest joints and avoiding positions of deformity

    c. Practicing vivid imagery and relaxation during difficult activities

    d. Applying heat before treatment and cold after range of motion

236. A patient in an automobile accident sustained an amputation of the right ring finger at the proximal interphalangeal joint. The patient complains of shocking pain when the finger touches most items and is concerned about returning to their job as an administrative secretary where more than 50% of the work involves typing on a computer. For the early phase of sensory reeducation, the OT should:
    a. Apply stimuli using light moving stroke to the affected area
    b. Use graded items including coarse to soft touch
    c. Wrap the digit in a light-weighted material or gauze
    d. Immerse the affected hand in a container of rice with various textured items

237. A patient can perform self-feeding with regular utensils. However, meal time must be monitored because of frequent coughing and fear of choking. Which is the BEST example of a statement that would document the patient's needs at mealtime?
    a. Patient requires minimal assist with self-feeding.
    b. Patient must be supervised during meals.
    c. Patient requires moderate assistance in self-feeding.
    d. Patient is dependent on caregiver for meals.

238. Which method would be the MOST effective for scar reduction caused by traumatic injuries or burns?
    a. Ace bandage
    b. Friction massage
    b. Compression
    d. Splinting

239. The OT is instructing a patient with a severe pulmonary condition in modifications of self-care skills. In order to monitor endurance for these basic activities, the OT should:
    a. Take the client's blood pressure often during the treatment session
    b. Have the patient rest every few minutes
    c. Stop the activity every few minutes, and have the client rate their level of fatigue
    d. Observe the breathing pattern of the patient while performing the activity

240. An occupational therapy program designed to teach an individual with cerebral palsy to compensate for poor handwriting would MOST likely involve the individual:
    a. Learning to type on a computer
    b. Practicing manipulation of nuts and bolts
    c. Practicing letter or shape formation
    d. Strengthening the intrinsic muscles of the hands

241. An OT is providing preprosthetic training to a young male with a left transhumeral amputation. Appropriate goals at this stage are to:
    a. Assist the person to explore new interests and leisure skills
    b. Practice balance activities in sitting and standing
    c. Promote skin healing and conditioning
    d. Assist in developing a new body image with prosthesis

242. An entry-level OT has a new job at an outpatient rehabilitation facility. The majority of diagnoses are conditions, such as tendonitis, fractures, overuse syndrome, and nerve compression injuries. The OT concludes that the primary frame of reference used to treat individuals at this facility is:
    a. Neurodevelopmental
    b. Cognitive
    c. Sensorimotor
    d. Biomechanical

243. During treatment, what approach should the OT follow when working with an individual that has a history of orthostatic hypotension?
    a. Keep the individual in a sitting position during therapy
    b. Assist the individual in slowly changing positions
    c. Place the individual in a reclined position during therapy
    d. In therapy, alternate between periods of work and rest

244. What is the MOST useful piece of adaptive equipment to use for an individual with tremors who has difficulty stabilizing and scooping food from a dish during mealtime?
    a. A non-skid mat
    b. A plate guard
    c. Swivel utensils
    d. A deep rimmed dish

245. An OT is working with an individual who has hypotonia in the upper extremities. An appropriate intervention for this deficit is to have the patient:
    a. Perform equilibrium activities
    b. Perform strengthening against gravity
    c. Perform alternate weight bearing and reaching activities
    d. Clasp both hands together and reach up to hit a ball

246. An individual who is confined to a wheelchair is unable to detect pain or pressure sensation. The OT should:
    a. Encourage the individual to transfer from wheelchair to a regular chair twice a day
    b. Suggest the individual use a pillow in the wheelchair

c. Require a family member to remind the individual to do pressure relief periodically

d. Educate on repositioning and how to check the skin for breakdown

247. You're working with an elderly patient who has cognitive difficulties and low vision issues. You decide that some simple crafts might be of use in treatment. Which of the following crafts would be the MOST appropriate to use?
a. Paint by number kit
b. Wood burning on a small wooden box lid
c. Copper tooling using recessed plastic forms
d. Coloring a poster

248. A client is choosing to work on tooling a leather wallet like one of his peers, but you know that his attention span is short and that doing such a project would likely set him up for failure. You decide to:
a. Let the client go ahead and try it, but tell the client that failure is likely, because the task is too difficult
b. Refuse to let the client work on the leather, because the client will just waste the materials
c. Tell the client that leatherwork is only for the skilled members of the group
d. Encourage the client to work a smaller piece (like a leather round) first to help him determine if the client likes the activity and if the client really wants to invest the time that it will take to complete the task

249. You are working with an adult patient in a day treatment program who wishes to become more assertive. Which of the following is the MOST appropriate goal for this patient's OT treatment?
a. Patient will tell others what they think
b. Patient will practice assertiveness skills twice a day
c. Patient will demonstrate improvement in assertiveness skills
d. Patient will demonstrate improvement in assertiveness skills by consistently voicing needs to their spouse, as they arise, for 2 weeks

250. An adult patient refuses to do any of the craft projects that you have in your clinic. Your best NEXT step would be to:
a. Ask what the patient enjoys doing and see if there is an alternative therapeutic activity that the patient might agree to engage in
b. Tell the patient to go back to the patient's room then and you will document that the patient refused
c. Ignore the patient, give attention to the other patients and see what happens
d. Tell the patient that a craft must be done because the doctor ordered it

251. Which of the following would MOST likely be part of an OT wellness and prevention program for older persons?
    a. ADL training
    b. Leisure planning education
    c. Education in effective communication with coworkers
    d. Reminiscence groups

252. An angry adolescent has a history of breaking things when angry and then feels guilty about it later. The BEST choice of activities for this client would be:
    a. Wedging clay to make a pot
    a. Knitting
    c. Painting a landscape picture
    d. A current events group

253. A patient has just joined your group. The patient worries about everything. Which of the following would the BEST activity for this patient in occupational therapy?
    a. Wedging clay to make a pot
    b. Assertiveness training
    c. Relaxation exercises
    d. Leatherwork

254. You have a patient who has memory problems. Which of the following would you MOST likely use?
    a. A written schedule of daily activities to remind the patient where they needs to be
    b. A daily log for the patient to express himself in writing
    c. A picture board to help communicate the patient's needs
    d. Flash cards to help the patient practice new words

255. You've been asked to evaluate a young adult who has previously been diagnosed with everything from schizophrenia to depression. This person has been able to live with minimal support in the community but struggles with maintaining a work role. You evaluate the client and note difficulty in the initiation of tasks but motivation to work and the desire to do a good job. Your recommendation would MOST likely include:
    a. A sheltered workshop environment providing a highly structured environment
    b. New efforts to independently find work in a fast food business
    c. A job coach in a supportive and structured work environment
    d. A less stressful work environment, where he can work more independently and at his own pace

256. An intervention that involves the provision of visual or auditory cues about physical processes, such as heart rate and muscle tension, that allows the patient to gain control over them is:
   a. Biofeedback
   b. Bradycardia
   c. Psychodynamics
   d. Psychodrama

257. Which of the following is a treatment used with depressed patients as a last resort and involves using electricity to cause a patient to have a seizure?
   a. Electroconvulsive therapy
   b. Insulin therapy
   c. Cryogenics
   d. Hypnosis

258. In working with a chronic pain patient, the OT would MOST likely:
   a. Suggest what medications would be best for the patient's pain
   b. Ignore the patient's complaints and tell them that "it is all in your head"
   c. Analyze the patient's occupational performance deficits and provide intervention to help the person regain control over their life
   d. Tell the patient that the only way that they will get better is if they exercise, even though they are in pain

259. In working with individuals who have been burned, the OT's role would be limited to:
   a. Treating wounds and avoiding contractures
   b. Evaluating any deficits in occupational performance, including psychosocial issues, and providing intervention that meets the patient's current occupational needs
   c. Fitting burn garments and maintaining ROM
   d. ROM and splinting as needed

260. Which of the following is the BEST example of a possible compensatory strategy a school-based OT may use to improve functional written communication for a student?
   a. Use of an adapted pencil grip
   b. Handwriting Without Tears
   c. Classroom based handwriting intervention group
   d. Keyboarding

261. Which of the following is the BEST example of inclusive or integrated school-based occupational therapy services?

   a.   The OT joins the teacher in assisting individual students to complete planned curriculum activities in the classroom.

   b.   The OT works with a small group of students in the back of the classroom.

   c.   The OT brings in fine motor activities for a student to complete at the desk.

   d.   The OT provides classroom staff with activities to follow through on with students during the week.

262. Which of the following interventions would be MOST reflective of direct occupational therapy services provided in an educational model as opposed to a medical setting?

   a.   Attending a field trip to assist a student who has difficulty transitioning cope in the unfamiliar environment

   b.   One-on-one sensory integration therapy

   c.   Pulling a student out to a separate room to practice fine motor activities

   d.   Adapting a worksheet for a student to complete in class

263. Which of the following potential sensory diet activities would be the MOST appropriate choice to provide proprioceptive input to for a preschool student?

   a.   Sitting on a therapy ball during fine motor craft activities

   b.   Rocking in a rocking chair while being read to

   c.   Sorting magnetic alphabet letters out of a bin of dried beans

   d.   Picking up weighted beanbags and placing them in a container during cleanup time

264. Which of the following is the BEST example of grading an activity to provide the "just right" challenge for a student receiving school-based occupational therapy?

   a.   The OT recommends that the classroom teacher provide the student with a copy of materials that are to be copied from the board to accommodate for visual perceptual difficulties.

   b.   The OT holds a cut and paste worksheet vertically to encourage the student to obtain wrist extension when cutting with scissors, enabling the student to better cut along a line.

   c.   The OT provides a pencil grip to cue the student to use a functional grasp for writing and drawing tasks.

   d.   The OT adapts a student's classroom seating to support better posture.

265. If you suspect a student diagnosed with seizure disorder or epilepsy is having a seizure during a therapy session, an important response would be:

   a.   Checking the student's mouth

   b.   Calling 911

    c.   Physically restraining any movements the student makes

    d.   Preventing the child from striking against any objects that may cause injury and allowing the seizure to conclude

266. Which of the following is NOT an example of appropriate consultation in school-based occupational therapy?

    a.   Discussing with a physical education teacher how to adapt activities to allow a student with cerebral palsy to participate

    b.   Recommending that a student use a pencil grip and incline writing surface to improve handwriting

    c.   Providing the classroom staff with sensory diet activities to help the student regulate the level of arousal

    d.   Providing therapy services in the natural classroom environment, rather than in a pull-out setting

267. Coordinated activities for a student with a disability that is an outcome-oriented process promoting movement from school to post-school activities; based in individual student needs, considering the student's preferences and interests; and including related services, instruction, community experiences, employment, and post-school living objectives, and if appropriate daily living skills and functional vocational evaluation (§300.29) MOST accurately describes which of the following?

    a.   School-based occupational therapy

    b.   Specially designed instruction (special education)

    c.   Individualized Education Plan

    d.   Transition services

268. The Wilbarger approach is a complementary treatment in sensory integration designed to address what?

    a.   Sensory defensiveness

    b.   Self-regulation

    c.   Sensory modulation

    d.   Vestibular processing

269. Which of the following would be the MOST appropriate activity to encourage development of in-hand manipulation skills?

    a.   Placing small pegs in a pegboard

    b.   Rotating a pencil in one hand to erase

    c.   Using a key to open a lock

    d.   Placing pegs in a pegboard

270. Which of the following might a school-based OT try during therapy with a student demonstrating visual discrimination difficulties?

    a.   Cutting out a significant part of a magazine picture and asking the child to try to determine what is missing

b. Using visually and tactilely stimulating activities, gradually increasing the sustained attention required for tasks
c. Playing a concentration game
d. Showing the student a group of objects, then asking the student to try to identify which one is missing after one has been removed from the group

271. Which of the following would be appropriate examples of assistive technology a school-based OT may recommend for handwriting?
a. Pencil grip
b. Inclined writing surface/slant board/easel
c. Dorsal hand weights
d. Word processor

Answers to Intervention Questions

1. b. The assessment is a time for the assessment team to utilize specific assessment tools to determine the needs of the child and with the help of the family establish treatment goals that are appropriate for the family. *Pediatric Occupational Therapy and Early Intervention* by Case-Smith

2. c. The most effective method for teaching parents intervention strategies is to use a learning style they are most comfortable with. These may be written handouts, videos, illustrations, or demonstration with the parents performing the activity with OT guidance and feedback. *Pediatric Occupational Therapy and Early Intervention* by Case-Smith

3. c. Rhythmic swinging calms the child while maintaining a level of alertness. This is an effective use of sensory preparation for activity. Combine this with rhythmic vocalization and deep pressure to help calm the child before engaging in an activity. The therapist must watch the child for response to the sensory preparation and gear input accordingly. *Occupational Therapy for Children* by Case-Smith

4. d. Reframing is utilized to promote understanding of the child and the child's disability. The OT provides information and reading material about the disability and helps interpret and explain delays. *Pediatric Occupational Therapy and Early Intervention* by Case-Smith

5. a. This is an example of adaptation. This is a change to the child's environment to allow for the child's highest level of participation in the home. Children that are sensory defensive frequently are agitated by tags on clothing. This eliminates that problem by adapting items in the environment. *Pediatric Occupational Therapy and Early Intervention* by Case-Smith

6. b. When providing touch to a child with sensory defensiveness, light and fleeting touches are often interpreted as painful and noxious. It is important to provide deep pressure in order to calm the sensory system. *Sensory Integration: Theory and Practice* by Bundy

7. b. The active movement allows the child to address postural needs as well as provide input into the vestibular system. This provides a calming and reorganizing effect to the sensory system and helps the child to focus on specific tasks. *Sensory Integration: Theory and Practice* by Bundy

8.   a.   The prone position is the best for facilitating neck and trunk extension whether on a ball, bolster, or wedge. *Occupational Therapy for Children* by Case-Smith

9.   c.   Neck flexion control is usually elicited by slowly raising the child from supine to sitting and lowering the child from sitting to supine. The OT gradually would lower the child backward from the sitting position until the child starts to lose head control. The OT then would assist the child to return to a sitting position. In this way neck flexor control is facilitated in both directions. *Occupational Theraphy for children* by Case-Smith

10. d.   The most common and effective position to place a child in is sitting, with attention given to the head and neck control, visual regard, and visual tracking. Although the child can be placed in the supine and sidelying positions, sitting is the most commonly used position. *Occupational Therapy for Children* by Case-Smith

11. c.   This is the best method to provide the child with the opportunity to play with toys independently and if the toy is dropped, the child will know how to find it. *Occupational Therapy for Children* by Case-Smith

12. a.   Using the surface to support the child's forearm and hand helps in the manipulation of the object. Using objects that roll or tiny objects are more difficult for the child. The child requires excellent tactile discrimination and fingertip control, so using these makes it more difficult. *Occupational Therapy for Children* by Case-Smith

13. b.   Children who are hyporesponsive seem to seek intensive stimulation. The child seeks large quantities of intense vestibular stimuli and although the child registers signs of pleasure, the input does not affect the nervous system to the extent that it does for most children. *Occupational Therapy for Children* by Case-Smith

14. a.   Children with cerebral palsy rarely become functional hand writers. Using conditional reasoning enables the OT to think about the long-term issues when planning for the short-term. As writing demands increase in the fourth and fifth grades, legibility and slow writing become greater issues. By beginning to learn the keyboard early, she can develop the word processing skills that she will need as writing assignments increase. Although she should be encouraged to practice handwriting, intervention emphasis is better placed on long-term solutions. *Occupational Therapy for Children* by Case-Smith

15. c. Providing a child with peel-off stickers is a compensatory strategy because it enables the child with limited drawing skills to make a picture with his peers. The other strategies listed, wearing a weighted vest and praising the child, are interventions to directly change the child's behavior or improve performance. *Occupational Therapy for Children* by Case-Smith

16. d. By placing a small weight on the patient's wrist, you are enhancing the proprioceptive input the patient receives when moving that arm. Therefore, you are using a strategy of augmented and individualized sensory cueing and feedback, which helps to improve performance. The other strategies involve adapting the activity so that it is easier for the patient to accomplish or so that the activity provides a "just right" challenge. Environment modifications entail improving the fit between child and environment. For promoting participation and preventing disability, it is important to educate other professionals and administrators and bring about a system change in the child's community. *Occupational Therapy for Children* by Case-Smith

17. a. Vestibular, tactile, and proprioceptive input are often used to increase or decrease a child's arousal and prepare the child to perform an activity. Linear swinging can organize a child and potentially improve attention to the activity. Rapid swinging can increase arousal and alertness. When a child performs a heavy work activity, they may feel more organized and calm to participate in other learning activities. Visual input through a computer game and auditory stimulation through listening to a story do not have powerful effects on arousal and are not used as preparatory activities. *Occupational Therapy for Children* by Case-Smith

18. b. To better attend and learn in the classroom, the OT recommends that the teacher modify the environment by decreasing distracting visual and auditory stimulation. In addition, the OT uses augmented and individualized sensory cueing and feedback by modifying handouts so that the amount of visual stimulation is reduced and the color and font size help maintain visual attention. These strategies help to improve attention and learning in the classroom. Using occupation as means and therapeutic use of self are used in one-on-one direct services and are not likely to be used. These strategies are used to improve specific performance (which in this case is not listed as a goal). *Occupational Therapy for Children* by Case-Smith

19. a. NDT is most effective in helping certain children, those with cerebral palsy, in developing specific motor skills. Performance

areas targeted when using NDT should be specifically and routinely measured to determine whether progress toward expected outcomes is satisfactory. NDT is not more effective for infants with spastic diplegia than infant stimulation. Experiments have shown that functional performance in children who receive intensive NDT is no different from the performance of children who receive regular occupational therapy that emphasized functional activities. *Occupational Therapy for Children* by Case-Smith

20. a. In inclusion, children receive services in their natural environment; when infants and toddlers and in the least restrictive environment. The natural environment can be the home or a child care center. It can be any setting where typical children play or are cared for. A special education classroom or a rehabilitation clinic are not examples of inclusion, because these are environments established specifically for individuals with disabilities. *Occupational Therapy for Children* by Case-Smith

21. b. Evidence-based practice includes deciding on an intervention strategy based on research findings, the OT's own experiences, and family priorities. Basing a decision about how to approach intervention solely on research findings without considering one's own experience and the family's priorities does not allow for consideration of all of the unique characteristics and needs of the child and family. *Occupational Therapy for Children* by Case-Smith

22. a. Cultural values are important to consider when working with children and their families. The OT should attempt to discern the family's view of disability, ideas about discipline, and values for independence versus intradependence. All of these can influence how accepting of intervention services the family is, what types of intervention strategies should be recommended, how to approach behavioral issues, and how to approach levels and types of services. *Occupational Therapy for Children* by Case-Smith

23. a. In contrast to the multidisciplinary team, the interdisciplinary team requires group synthesis. Professionals collaborate in planning intervention and service delivery. In multidisciplinary teams, members function relatively autonomously and each member is respected for his or her expertise in a defined practice area. Members have a good understanding of other professionals' scopes of practice and rely on these team members to fulfill their roles. Neither interdisciplinary nor

multidisciplinary teams always have consensus. *Occupational Therapy for Children* by Case-Smith

24. a. Physical therapists provide intervention to improve motor skills, mobility, balance, and coordination. They assist in equipment design, fabrication, and fitting. For specific children, they may be involved in burn and wound care or exercise to improve cardiopulmonary endurance. Speech and language pathologists are the primary professionals to assess for and train in augmentative communication. School psychologists and teachers are the primary professions to assess social skills. They also are the primary professions to design interventions to promote social skills, although other professionals, including occupational therapists, support children's development of social skills. *Occupational Therapy for Children* by Case-Smith

25. d. There are 17 early intervention services identified in Part C of IDEA. They are as follows: (1) family training, counseling, home visits, (2) special instruction, (3) speech therapy, (4) hearing therapy, (5) occupational therapy, (6) physical therapy, (7) psychological sessions, (8) service coordination, (9) medical diagnosis or evaluation, (10) early identification, screening, and assessment, (11) health program, (12) social work, (13) vision, (14) nursing, (15) nutrition, (16) assistive technology devices and instructions, and (17) transportation and financial counseling. Of the services listed in the question, only medical care and surgery are not listed as provided services in IDEA. *Occupational Therapy for Children* by Case-Smith

26. a. As a first step, the team must develop a comprehensive description of the problem, including individual and environmental factors that influence the issue, and they should define the problem clearly and objectively. The team members should then make a commitment to solving the problem. Making a decision and developing a plan for achieving the solution based on that decision and identifying as many strategies as possible to reduce barriers and increase supports should not occur first but should follow a discussion in which the problem is clearly identified and analyzed. *Occupational Therapy for Children* by Case-Smith

27. b. The role of a nurse in early intervention includes diagnosing and treating health problems in children and families; screening and assessing the psychologic, physiologic, and developmental characteristics of the child and family for early identification, referral, and intervention; planning and coordinating with the family and interdisciplinary team; providing intervention

to the family to improve the child's and family's health and developmental status; and evaluating the effectiveness of the nursing care provided. Providing treatment to increase joint function, muscle strength, mobility, and endurance are part of a physical therapist's role. *Occupational Therapy for Children* by Case-Smith

28. a. In transdisciplinary services, one member of the team generally provides direct services and the others provide consultation to that individual. In this case the nurse provides direct services to the family and the OT consults with the nurse. *Occupational Therapy for Children* by Case-Smith

29. c. Maslow's hierarchy of basic human needs is believed to follow a longitudinal sequence beginning with basic physiologic needs, such as food, water, and air, and ending with the need for self-actualization. When basic lower-level needs are not being met, it is proposed that higher order tasks or abilities (e.g., intellect), which are ranked higher on the hierarchy, are compromised. *Occupational Theraphy for Children* by Case-Smith

30. b. The dynamic systems approach is similar to some of the occupational therapy theories that focus on person, environment, and occupation relationships. *Occupational Therapy for Children* by Case-Smith

31. a. According to the social cognitive theory introduced by Bandura, there are two stages in learning: acquisition and performance. During acquisition, a child observes the behavior of others and determines the consequences, and these observations are stored in memory for later use. *Occupational Therapy for Children* by Case-Smith

32. b. This strategy would enable her to concentrate better without distraction and help her develop better relations with her peers in the classroom. *Occupational Therapy for Children* by Case-Smith

33. b. At the age of 4 months, infants can lift the head to visualize activities in the room. By 6 months, they roll sequentially to progress across the room. They can also move side to side on the forearms, then the hands, and can lift an arm to grasp a toy. Although they cannot sit erect and unsupported for a long time, they sit alone by propping forward on the arms, using a wide base of support with the legs flexed. At 7 months, they can crawl forward. When they are 8–9 months, they can sit erect and unsupported. *Occupational Therapy for Children* by Case-Smith

34. b. A 5-year-old child develops a mature, dynamic tripod grasp. In this grasp pattern the pencil is held in the tips of the radial fingers and is moved using finger movement. By controlling the pencil using individual finger movements, the child can make letters and small forms. *Occupational Therapy for Children* by Case-Smith

35. c. OTs should refrain from making definitive statements about the future, as long-range predictions about when the child will achieve a certain milestone or level of independence are always speculative. However, parents feel frustrated when they are told that the future cannot be predicted. The OT should therefore help parents understand the range of possibilities by telling them about the continuum of services for older children and young adults in the community. *Occupational Therapy for Children* by Case-Smith

36. d. The OT needs to help them build their problem-solving skills. When others direct parents, they become more dependent. However, when parents successfully solve a problem, they become empowered to act independently in daily decision-making. The OT should also focus on their internal and external control, self-esteem, and social skills and take note of their learning styles and abilities so as to better instruct them on the care for their child. The OT should not make decision for them, because this would decrease their sense of empowerment. A decision made for them is one that they would probably not implement with and may resent. *Occupational Therapy for Children* by Case-Smith

37. b. To help the parents cope with the situation, they need to develop friendships with other parents experiencing similar circumstances. This way, the parents can provide emotional support to one another and assist each other in resolving specific dilemmas in daily routines. IDEA also requires that children have access to normal environments. Meeting with church groups and talking with park and recreation may help identify ways community activities can be more inclusive. *Occupational Therapy for Children* by Case-Smith

38. b. GMFM is a criterion-referenced test that measures the components of a gross motor activity that a child with cerebral palsy can accomplish. It provides the OT with the information necessary for designing intervention programs. SFA is used to evaluate the child's performance of occupational roles in the context of daily life, specifically in tasks that support participation in the academic

and social aspects. It is used with children of an elementary school program, so the child is too young for this assessment. SIPT is a standardized test used to help identify difficulties in the different areas of sensory functioning. MAP is used frequently for preschool domain screening purposes not for intervention programming. *Occupational Therapy for Children* by Case-Smith

39. c. Biofeedback can provide the needed feedback to the child about successful and unsuccessful muscle activation or positioning. It increases the child's motivation and improves the head control in sitting and prone positions. *Occupational Therapy for Children* by Case-Smith

40. d. Although feedback is essential to learning, it is found to be detrimental if given profusely. Intermittent feedback earlier on and decreasing feedback as skill develops would be ideal. Second, movements should not be repeated over an extended period of time as it leads to blocked practice. There should be an intermittent and random schedule. Third, handling may cause ineffective motor learning as the child depends on the assistance or handling may prevent errors and impair learning. *Occupational Therapy for Children* by Case-Smith

41. b. Activities that require stabilization with grasp should be encouraged, because such activities are beginning to be used and could be developed to be more consistent, which would help her accomplish a variety of functional tasks. The OT also can encourage symmetric bilateral hand use in order to promote increased awareness of the left arm and improved ability to hold and carry objects with both hands together. Activities that require stabilization without grasp may be able to be accomplished if the activities do not require the hand to be open. Simultaneous bilateral manipulation skills will be inappropriate. However, intervention to support the increased use of in-hand manipulation skills may be appropriate, but skills that are easier than complex rotation with stabilization will need to be the focus. Because this patient is still fisting with the left hand and can only use a palmar grasp, emphasis on a pincer grasp would present too great a challenge. *Occupational Therapy for Children* by Case-Smith

42. d. When using a hand splint with a child with spasticity, frequent follow-up is necessary to check the fit, make modifications if necessary, and verify comfort. In addition, follow-up is necessary to determine if other abnormal patterns of movement

are emerging when the hand posture is changed by the splint. *Occupational Therapy for Children* by Case-Smith

43. a. According to the motor learning theory, the OT assists the child in acquiring specific motor learning skills through structure and feedback and provides him or her with structured practice to refine the skills. Although the behavioral theory also involves specific feedback, it emphasizes tasks or functional activities that involve more than motor components. *Occupational Therapy for Children* by Case-Smith

44. c. Because the finger pad grasp pattern is important for precise placement and as a basis for mature release, this is a key are of focus in intervention. In addition, bilateral skills need to be addressed, but skills that involve stabilizing with one hand would be the priority, rather than symmetrical bilateral skills, because these skills do not require differentiation of the actions of the two hands, which is an area of difficulty that this child demonstrates. *Occupational Therapy for Children* by Case-Smith

45. b. Providing verbal cueing for strategies to use in performing skills and providing a demonstration of skills is useful in the case of children who possess some basic in-hand manipulation skills. For children who possess no in-hand manipulation skills, the OT may encourage the manipulation of objects between two hands and encourage the use of support surfaces to assist in object manipulation. Use of these strategies can help children begin to move the fingers actively over object surfaces. *Occupational Therapy for Children* by Case-Smith

46. c. Classic sensory integration therapy is applied on an individual basis and the emphasis is on the inner drive of the child. Individual therapy is the most intense form of intervention and it allows the OT to adjust therapeutic activities moment by moment in relation to the individual child's interest in the activity or response in a sensory experience. Group therapy is sometimes used as a transition from individual therapy so that the child can apply new skills in the social context with less intensive support. Consultation is an indirect form of intervention. Helping the family members and teachers who come in contact with the child understand the problem can be an effective way of helping the child. *Occupational Therapy for Children* by Case-Smith

47. b. Occupational therapy is not expected to cure sensory integrative dysfunction. Parents need to know that the aim is

to improve the sensory integrative functions and the quality of life of a child. They should try to help the child in learning compensatory skills that will minimize the effects of the problems. Giving the parents a tentative time period based on the severity of the problem is not possible because occupational therapy does not "cure" sensory integrative disorders. Also, informing the parents that there is no fixed time period could create anxiety. In such a situation, OTs need to counsel the parents and explain the problem and the effects it will have on their lives. *Occupational Therapy for Children* by Case-Smith

48. b. The behavior observed indicates that the child might have dyspraxia and is displaying problems with ideation. Being unable to complete a simple puzzle, not being spontaneous during play, and wandering aimlessly when left alone are typical responses observed in dyspraxia. Hence the child might have problems with ideation. The child may appear clumsy and awkward, but the inability to do simple things cannot be ignored. In somatodyspraxia, directionality of movement is disturbed and the child may find it difficult to relate the body to physical objects in environmental space. There is also difficulty in imitating actions of others. Problems with bilateral integration and sequencing are characterized by poor bilateral coordination and difficulty in sequencing actions. *Occupational Therapy for Children* by Case-Smith

49. b. A splint with the palmar bar proximal to the distal palmar crease will permit metacarpophalangeal flexion and allows the fingers to be free for greater use of the hand while providing support to the affected wrist. A wrist cock-up splint will generally accomplish this goal. *Introduction to Splinting: A Clinical Reasoning and Problem Solving Approach* by Coppard and Lohman

50. a. The resting hand splint has three primary purposes: to immobilize for rest, to promote functional alignment, and to minimize or prevent further deformity. It is often the splint of choice with inflamed swollen joints and improper joint alignment as seen in arthritis. *Introduction to Splinting: A Clinical Reasoning and Problem Solving Approach* by Coppard and Lohman

51. c. Perspiration is related to temperature regulation or the exchange of air to the underlying skin. A splint with perforations and greater permeability will allow greater air flow. *Introduction to Splinting: A Clinical Reasoning and Problem Solving Approach* by Coppard and Lohman

52. d. The NDT approach advocates the use of the reflex-inhibiting patterns to inhibit spasticity. Finger and thumb abduction are key to controlling spasticity by facilitating extensor muscle tone and inhibiting flexor tone. *Introduction to Splinting: A Clinical Reasoning and Problem Solving Approach* by Coppard and Lohman

53. a. A boutonniere deformity is characterized by rupture or stretch in the lateral bands that leads to a flexion deformity of the proximal interphalangeal joint and hyperextension of the distal interphalangeal joint. In order to correct this type of deformity with a splint, both the proximal interphalangeal and the distal interphalangeal joints should be placed in full extension. *Occupational Therapy for Physical Dysfunction* by Trombly and Radomski

54. c. The focus of occupational therapy with burns in the early stages is to prevent deformity by keeping structures involved aligned. Concerns should also focus on promoting integrity and mobility and preventing the shortening of ligaments, joint capsule, muscles, and tendons. *Introduction to Splinting: A Clinical Reasoning and Problem Solving Approach* by Coppard and Lohman

55. b. Functional hand positioning with wide strapping or compression wrapping is useful for controlling edema. In this case, straps on a splint will cause pocketing of fluid in areas of the extremity. Because edema status changes quickly, this must be monitored closely for splint adjustments. *Introduction to Splinting: A Clinical Reasoning and Problem Solving Approach* by Coppard and Lohman

56. c. If there are no other fitting issues, a strategy to solve the problem of pressure over the styloid process is to spot heat and stretch splinting material over the affected area. Discarding the splint is not necessary if no other conformity issues are identified. Placing padding over the area reduces space and thus may actually increase pressure, and change in the wearing schedule does not address the problem. *Introduction to Splinting: A Clinical Reasoning and Problem Solving Approach* by Coppard and Lohman

57. d. One precaution for patients with hip surgery is to avoid flexing the hip greater than 90%. To reduce hip flexion when sitting, patients with hip replacement surgery are often instructed to use a raised toilet seat. *Occupational Therapy for Physical Dysfunction* by Trombly and Radomski

58. a. A person with a hip fracture should avoid any activity, such as shoe tying, which could potentially cause hip flexion to 90

degrees or greater. Such a position could actually undo the benefits of the surgical procedure. *Occupational Therapy for Physical Dysfunction* by Trombly and Radomski

59. a. An individual with a T1 spinal cord injury has innervations of all the upper extremity musculature, including the intrinsics and partial innervations of erector spinae muscles for weak trunk balance, and is generally able to operate a manual wheelchair. *Occupational Therapy for Physical Dysfunction* by Trombly and Radomski

60. b. Persons with spinal cord lesions at T6 and above are at risk for autonomic dysreflexia, which can occur as a result of the individual being overheated, stressed, in pain, or having urinary and bowel complications. Autonomic dysreflexia is considered a medical emergency, and symptoms include hypertension, pounding headache, sweating, flushing, pupil constriction, and nasal congestion. *Conditions in Occupational Therapy* by Atchinson

61. c. If there are no other complications, a minimally displaced fracture should be immobilized for short period (about 1 week) and then active controlled ROM should begin to minimize stiffness. Begin weaning the patient from the sling as active mobilization increases. *Hand Rehabilitation: A Quick Reference Guide and Review* by Weiss and Falkenstein

62. c. Abnormal resistance to passive movement or increased tone is the result of a stretch reflex. When a stretch reflex is triggered, this can lead to active tension of a muscle at any point during the ROM arc. This reflex may also create a significant force that pulls the wrist and fingers into an abnormal shortened resting state, such as a flexor synergy pattern. An antispasticity splint is designed to provide a sustained consistent stretch to spastic muscles, thus facilitating a more relaxed state in the muscle. Once the muscle relaxes, functional movement can be facilitated. *Introduction to Splinting: A Clinical Reasoning and Problem Solving Approach* by Coppard and Lohman

63. b. An intrinsic plus position promotes the position of digital metacarpophalangeal flexion and interphalangeal extension that maintains the length of the collateral ligaments and volar plate. This position is often preferred when severe injury has the potential to lead to deformity, such as in the case of tissue loss or burns. The intrinsic plus position is also called the antideformity position. *Occupational Therapy for Physical Dysfunction* by Trombly and Radomski

64. b. A weighted cuff on the wrist can be used to dampen the effects of intention tremors or uncoordinated movements. The resistance provided by the cuff may help to provide some stability, enabling the individual to exert more control. *Occupational Therapy for Physical Dysfunction* by Trombly and Radomski

65. b. Children with ADHD will have both attention deficits and deficits with motor function, such as lethargy or clumsiness. Structured repetitive activities that address both motor acuity and captures may capture the child's attention while addressing coordination issues. *Occupational Therapy for Children* by Case-Smith

66. d. For a child who will eventually use Braille or need their hands for constant communication, the importance of early perceptual and tactile training is essential. An activity that encourages the use of the fingers is appropriate because this is a similar method used for reading Braille. Also, the scratch activity provides constant repetitive stimulation to the finger tips that would assist in decreasing tactile defensiveness. *Occupational Therapy for Children* by Case-Smith

67. c. The patient with a T4 spinal cord lesion would need to have a wheelchair with removable arms to perform sliding transfers. Clients who are unstable or confused would need support. *Conditions in Occupational Therapy* by Hansen and Atchinson

68. c. Children with gravitational insecurity usually show pleasure at receiving vestibular stimulation including having the head radically tilted in different planes. Playing on the swings or suspended equipment provides the movement or vestibular stimulation that helps the child feel more secure and safe. *Occupational Therapy for Children* by Case-Smith

69. c. Children with sensory integrative deficits would benefit from a program that provides organized tactile and proprioceptive input thorough sensorimotor activities. Organized sensorimotor input promotes sensory organization and modulation. *Occupational Therapy for Children* by Case-Smith

70. b. A boutonniere deformity is typically characterized by PIP joint flexion and DIP joint hyperextension. To correct this position, the therapist must place the affected digit in the opposite positions: PIP extension and DIP extension. *Introduction to Splinting: A Clinical Reasoning and Problem Solving Approach* by Coppard and Lohman

71. a. The OT should apply a hand to the child's chin from front or side to promote chin tuck and provide stability to jaw. One finger places pressure through the front of the chin and another provides support for the jaw. The fingers under the jaw prevent wide jaw excursions and assist in promoting the appropriate tongue movements. *Occupational Therapy for Children* by Case-Smith

72. d. One standard precaution with persons who undergo hip replacement surgery is to avoid positions and activities that would require bending the hip pass 90 degrees. Sitting on a regular toilet seat would compromise the surgery and outcome. An elevated toilet seat will help alleviate this problem. *Occupational Therapy for Physical Dysfunction* by Trombly and Radomski

73. d. A common reaction of a person in pain is to try to exert control by frustrating the pain program and proving to the team that the pain is indeed present and severe. Success of a pain program is aimed at changing the perception of the individual and having insight into his or her problems. Constant complaining should be ignored. The persons involved with the patient should identify the prize or goal the person is willing to work toward and reinforce health behavior that moves toward that goal. *Basic Rehabilitation Techniques: A Self Instructional Guide* by Sine, Liss, Roush, Holcomb, and Wilson

74. c. A person with a C5 spinal cord lesion has innervation of the deltoid, rotator cuff muscles, biceps, and brachioradialis. The triceps muscle, used for push ups, is not innervated at this level. Pressure relief is achieved through weight shifting techniques, such as using the biceps or elbow flexion and hooking the arm around the arm rest of the wheelchair. In the supine position, the person may use arm rail on the bed to assist in rolling from side to side. *Basic Rehabilitation Techniques: A Self Instructional Guide* by Sine, Liss, Roush, Holcomb, and Wilson

75. b. A progressive mobilization program should focus on getting the patient out of bed and keeping the patient out of bed and engaged in activities that are as close to normal as possible. Moving to the bathroom for ADLs will allow increased mobility to the appropriate setting for performing self-care. *Basic Rehabilitation Techniques: A Self Instructional Guide* by Sine, Liss, Roush, Holcomb, and Wilson

76. d. With limited ROM of the forearm, swivel utensils adjust so that as the food is carried from plate to mouth, the utensil compensates for the lack of pronation and supination. *Basic*

Rehabilitation Techniques: A Self Instructional Guide by Sine, Liss, Roush, Holcomb, and Wilson

77. a. With limited ROM and pain in the shoulders or elbows, lightweight, long-handled adapted equipment that can be positioned at the desired angle is preferred. *Basic Rehabilitation Techniques: A Self Instructional Guide* by Sine, Liss, Roush, Holcomb, and Wilson

78. a. Patients with emphysema will have limited ability to perform ADLs because of dyspnea. Many patients breathe shallowly and quickly. Breathing patterns should be noted when performing ADLs. In pulmonary rehabilitation, one way to monitor oxygen saturation is with the use of a pulse oximeter. Using a pulse oximeter, hypoxemia is recognized at 90% oxygen saturation. *Occupational Therapy for Physical Dysfunction* by Trombly and Radomski

79. d. The biomechanical approach emphasizes intervention programs that address musculoskeletal elements, such as ROM, strength, and endurance problems affecting occupation. *Occupational Therapy for Physical Dysfunction* by Trombly

80. d. In transdisciplinary service models, one member of the team generally provides direct services and the others provide consultation to that individual. In this case, the nurse provides direct services to the family and the OT consults with the nurse. *Occupational Therapy for Children* by Case-Smith

81. b. The emergence of drawing skills reflects both cognitive abilities and fine motor skills in children. By 4 years of age, children can identify the parts of a body, name them correctly, and represent them on a two-dimensional surface. This demonstrates their ability to select salient features and represent them on a two-dimensional surface. *Occupational Therapy for Children* by Case-Smith

82. b. Using a dynamic tripod grasp pattern, the pencil is held in the tips of the radial fingers and is moved using finger movement. This allows the child to exert greater control over the writing instrument using individual finger movements. A child usually develops first a static and then a dynamic tripod grasp around the age of 5; this enables the child to become more proficient at making letters and small forms. *Occupational Therapy for Children* by Case-Smith

83. c. Although all of the interventions can be used to facilitate head and postural control, biofeedback is a method that allows the individual to learn "cause and effect" by providing the feedback for successful and unsuccessful attempts. Thus, it can increase the child's motivation and improve head control in sitting and prone positions. *Occupational Therapy for Children* by Case-Smith

84. b. Children who lack antigravity muscle strength and stability can be provided stability through blocking or fixing certain joints, particularly in weight-bearing positions. *Occupational Therapy for Children* by Case-Smith

85. d. The Medical Restorative Model provides short-term intervention to persons who require long-term maintenance and episodic restorative services to maximize their level of functional independence. Persons with degenerative conditions or those that might loose function because of aging problems, such as dementia and Alzheimer's, often benefit from restorative interventions. *Occupational Therapy in Community-Based Practice Setting* by Scaffa

86. a. Purse lip breathing technique is helpful when shortness of breath occurs. Technique: the person inhales deeply through nose, purses the lips as though whistling, and very slowly exhales through the lips. *Quick Reference to Occupational Therapy* by Reed; *Occupational Therapy Practice Skills for Physical Dysfunction* by Pedretti and Early

87. c. Patients with perceptual dysfunction do best with as many tactile cues as possible paired with verbal cues if appropriate. *Vision, Perception and Cognition* by Zoltan

88. b. A client with a C4 injury would have innervation of the muscles controlling the head, neck, and diaphragm and would be the most appropriate choice for these activities. *Occupational Therapy for Physical Dysfunction* by Trombly and Radomski

89. d. A client with a C6 injury would have control of the head, neck, diaphragm, deltoids, biceps, and wrist extensors, giving the client enough function to complete the activities. *Occupational Therapy for Physical Dysfunction* by Trombly and Radomski

90. c. This would be the best choice because it can be mounted to the wheelchair and will allow for the most ease of movement in a safe manner. *Occupational Therapy Practice Skills for Physical Dysfunction* by Pedretti and Early

91. b. The loops would be the best. The client would be unable to use a trigger reacher and the standard dressing stick because the client does not have a functional grasp. The universal cuff would be of no benefit to grip and don pants and could only be used for closure with an additional device (button hook/zipper pull). *Occupational Therapy Practice Skills for Physical Dysfunction* by Pedretti and Early

92. b. An individual with this level injury would be able to use head, neck, diaphragm, deltoids, and biceps, but would not have wrist extensors that would allow for greater independence in self-care. An individual with a C4 injury would require greater assistance with dressing. *Occupational Therapy Practice Skills for Physical Dysfunction* by Pedretti and Early

93. c. Although all of these activities may seem appropriate for someone with a vision field deficit, the balloon batting would allow the individual with the most opportunities for presentation of items into the involved visual field versus the intact visual field, and encourage the person to increase the intact visual field usage. *Occupational Therapy Practice Skills for Physical Dysfunction* by Pedretti and Early

94. b. The motor control model is specifically designed and applicable to individuals with central nervous system dysfunction. This model includes the four treatment approaches by Rood, Brunnstom, Knott, and Voss and Bobath. Although the other models may contain elements that are beneficial for those who have central nervous system damage, only the motor control model would provide the comprehensive approach that is most beneficial for this population. *Occupational Therapy Practice Skills for Physical Dysfunction* by Pedretti and Early

95. c. When ascending or descending stairs, the cane should move with the painful/weak leg. Specifically, when ascending the stairs the leg without the cane should move first, allowing the weak leg and cane to bear the weight for only a short amount of time until the strong leg is able to provide the needed stability. *Occupational Therapy Practice Skills for Physical Dysfunction* by Pedretti and Early

96. c. The use of physical agent modalities is not consistent with the rehabilitation approach. Physical agent modalities are considered adjunct to therapy and in occupational therapy should be followed by functional activities. *Occupational Therapy Practice Skills for Physical Dysfunction* by Pedretti and Early

97. d. This is the only activity that will allow the client to address both issues as well as facilitate rehearsal from the rehab team. *Occupational Therapy for Physical Dysfunction* by Trombly and Radomski

98. a. Ideomotor apraxia is defined by Zoltan as the inability to imitate gestures or perform purposeful motor tasks on command, even though the patient fully understands the idea or concept of the task. The others would describe different difficulties for the client. *Vision, Perception and Cognition* by Zoltan

99. d. Although all of these are important, the time spent in posttraumatic amnesia has the biggest impact on functional activities. *Occupational Therapy for Physical Dysfunction* by Trombly and Radomski

100. b. Although a universal cuff, dressing loops, and a button hook may assist someone with a stroke, the person would be more likely to use the uninvolved hand or leg to complete tasks more easily as opposed to using the involved extremity with a device. *Stroke Rehabilitation a Functional-Based Approach* by Gillen and Burkhardt

101. a. Brushing would be considered to be facilitatory in this case and all the others would be inhibitory. *Occupational Therapy for Physical Dysfunction* by Trombly and Radomski

102. a. As an entry level OT, your most appropriate role on the team would be in the oral preparatory and oral phases. With additional training and continuing education, the OT could also be involved with the other phases as well. *Occupational Therapy Practice Skills for Physical Dysfunction* by Pedretti and Early

103. a. The use of gravity is the most common principle, with the other methods listed being less appropriate. *Occupational Therapy for Physical Dysfunction* by Trombly and Radomski

104. d. Clients with CVAs do not do well with assistive equipment because of perceptual problems. Adapted techniques— teaching a client to do something in a different way—has proven to be more effective. This is true because the adaptive equipment is unfamiliar to the client and the actual function may be difficult to comprehend when given to someone that may have cognitive or perceptual difficulties. Lightweight or weighted items would be appropriate to use with other neurologic clients for other reasons, but would not be

appropriate for CVAs. *Stroke Rehabilitation: A Function-Based Approach* by Gillen and Burkhardt

105. a. Clients with Broca's aphasia have slow labored speech with some apraxia also noted, but they have good receptive language skills unless it is too rapid or lengthy. *Occupational Therapy Practice Skills for Physical Dysfunction* by Pedretti and Early

106. b. Individuals with left hemispheric lesions usually do retain scanning skills, and the comments about right hemispheric lesions are not always true. *Occupational Therapy for Physical Dysfunction* by Trombly and Radomski

107. d. Upper extremity weight bearing is the only one of the choices that will actually improve the stability. *Occupational Therapy for Children* by Case-Smith

108. c. The adaptive response is the response that is made when presented with a situation that allows the individual success with the situation. *Occupational Therapy for Children* by Case-Smith

109. a. The just right challenge is one that provides the positive change but one that is not too difficult nor too easy for the child *Occupational Therapy for Children* by Case-Smith

110. b. The clinical observations section would include the actual performance of motor skills and components of the child during the evaluation process. *Occupational Therapy for Children* by Case-Smith

111. b. Body image is the way that we appear to ourselves. It is the part of us that makes us feel tall, short, small, large, and so forth. *Occupational Therapy for Children* by Case-Smith

112. d. Although all of the answer choices may improve handwriting, only the vertical writing surface will help to develop the grip and direction during handwriting. *Occupational Therapy for Children* by Case-Smith

113. c. In the assessment portion of the SOAP note, the therapist indicates progress in treatment or explains the failure to progress as quickly as anticipated. *Documentation Manual for Writing SOAP Notes in Occupational Therapy* by Borcherding

114. c. The patient's observations about the right upper extremity are most pertinent to this treatment session, because it relates to the entire

session. Nursing's comments are important but do not belong in the S section. The S section is usually reserved for the patient's comments. *Documentation Manual for Writing SOAP Notes in Occupational Therapy* by Borcherding

115. c.   The emphasis is on the performance component and the functional application, not the specific media used in the treatment. Many third-party payers also want to see the amount of time per Current Procedural Terminology code charged. *Documentation Manual for Writing SOAP Notes in Occupational Therapy* by Borcherding

116. b.   Choice (a) is the problem list, which goes in A; (c) is a justification for further treatment, which goes in A; (d) is what occured in treatment, which goes in O. *Documentation Manual for Writing SOAP Notes in Occupational Therapy* by Borcherding

117. a.   Although some of the responses are sound care measures, the most important reason to apply a splint on a child is to improve function. Irritation and pressure from wearing the splint would definitely affect the child's hand function. *Hand Function in the Child* by Henderson and Pehoski

118. d.   Parents have a right to know what you are doing with their child and most parents want to learn effective ways to handle their infant; family support is an integral part of therapeutic intervention strategies. *Occupational Therapy for Children* by Case-Smith

119. d.   Hearing aids, eyeglasses, and night lights are equipment or interventions used to improve functional performance. *Functional Performance in Older Adults* by Bonder and Wagner

120. a.   Strategic placement of the index and middle fingers place pressure through the front of the chin to promote chin tuck, and a thumb on a child's cheek allows stable manipulation of the mandible for chewing. *Occupational Therapy for Children* by Case-Smith

121. d.   A kyphotic posture is one with a curvature in the thoracic region, making donning pullover garments difficult. *Functional Performance in Older Adults* by Bonder and Wagner

122. a.   To compensate for decreased taste and smell associated with aging, the choice of foods should emphasize appearance and texture for appeal. *Aging: The Health Care Challenge* by Lewis

123. b.   Ergonomic interventions generally fall into one of four categories: engineering controls, work practice controls, administrative controls, and personal protective equipment. Stretch breaks, proper work techniques, employee conditioning, and job coaching are considered work practice controls. *Ergonomics and the Management of Musculoskeletal Disorders* by Sanders

124. a.   Ergonomic interventions generally fall into one of four categories: engineering controls, work practice controls, administrative controls, and personal protective equipment. Modifying workstations, suspending power hand tools, modifying operating controls, and seating are all considered engineering controls. *Ergonomics and the Management of Musculoskeletal Disorders* by Sanders

125. c.   Ergonomic interventions generally fall into one of four categories: engineering controls, work practice controls, administrative controls, and personal protective equipment. Reducing production rates, limiting overtime, recommending rest breaks, increasing the number of employees assigned to a task, job rotation, and equipment maintenance are all examples of administrative controls. *Ergonomics and the Management of Musculoskeletal Disorders* by Sanders

126. c.   Engineering controls are considered the most effective strategy for preventing or avoiding work-related injuries by eliminating the risk factors altogether. *Ergonomics and the Management of Musculoskeletal Disorders* by Sanders

127. b.   The inferior pincer grasp is characterized by thumb adduction and emerging opposition. When a child uses this grasp, they hold the object proximal to the pads of the finger. This grasp is typically seen between 8–9 months of age. The radial digital grasp typically emerges around the same time as the inferior pincer grasp. The raking grasp is generally seen between 7–8 months of age, and the three-jaw chuck is typically first seen between 10–12 months of age. *Hand Function in the Child* by Henderson and Pehoski

128. d.   A spherical grasp is useful for holding a ball or other round objects and turning a door knob. A spherical grasp is characterized by stabilization of the wrist, abduction of the fingers, flexion at the MCP and IP joints, and stability of the longitudinal arch. The fourth and fifth digits are flexed and cup the item and hold it close to the palm, which differs from their positions in the cylindrical grasp. *Developmental and*

Functional Hand Grasps by Edwards, Buckland, and McCoy-Powlen

129. c. Placing the thumb and the middle finger in the loops of the scissors with the index finger resting against the shaft of the handle is the correct way to hold scissors. By holding scissors in this manner, the index finger can guide the cutting, as well as provide strength and stability. If the scissors are held correctly, the child will activate the same muscles needed to manipulate a pencil with a mature grip. *Occupational Therapy for Children* by Case-Smith

130. a. Visual discrimination is the ability to detect features of stimuli for recognition, matching, and categorization. The specific visual discrimination abilities require the ability to note similarities and differences among forms and symbols with increasing complexity and then relate these back to information previously stored in long-term memory. Many preacademic and academic tasks rely on visual discrimination abilities. *Occupational Therapy for Children* by Case-Smith

131. d. The speech and language pathologist should position herself directly in front of the child so that the child does not have to turn or lift her head. Asking the child to turn or lift her head for any length of time will likely cause the child to go into a pattern of extension, making phonation difficult. *Handling the Young Child with Cerebral Palsy at Home* by Finnie

132. b. Only option (b) would support the child's goal of doffing his own shoes while maintaining an optimal and efficient position. The other options would place the child in an inefficient flexion pattern, making it difficult to maintain postural stability and use his legs, arms, and hands functionally. *Handling the Young Child with Cerebral Palsy at Home* by Finnie

133. c. By placing her index finger in a horizontal position between the child's upper lip and nose and providing firm and continuous pressure, the teacher will assist the child in mouth closing and allow the child ample time to swallow. Repeated use of this intervention will promote spontaneous mouth-closure and spontaneous swallowing. *Handling the Young Child with Cerebral Palsy at Home* by Finnie

134. b. According to traditional NDT, weight-bearing and weight-shifting activities provide stability and alignment in the active extremity and contribute to the development of control. By providing the child with opportunities to weight bear and

weight shift on the elbows and hands, the OT is hoping to help the child develop the requisite skills necessary for reach. *Pediatric Occupational Therapy and Early Intervention* by Case-Smith

135. c. The single switch is usually the best device to first introduce a child to in terms of technological devices and access systems. Initially the single switch can be connected to a toy. By playing with the switch toy the child can develop basic skills, such as object permanence and cause and effect. The child will also learn that he can control his surroundings. *Pediatric Occupational Therapy and Early Intervention* by Case-Smith

136. b. The key to treatment of oral hypersensitivity and aversion is to provide graded sensory input. Treatment should begin at the level at which the child is comfortable, and then slowly build to a point just below the threshold for elicitation of a hyper-sensitive-aversive response. *Pediatric Occupational Therapy and Early Intervention* by Case-Smith

137. a. Playing a matching game would address the child's underlying need: the ability to perceive the differences between letters. Both activities emphasize visual discrimination, or the ability to detect features of stimuli for recognition, matching, and categorization. *Occupational Therapy for Children* by Case-Smith

138. d. The use of a spacer, such as a penny, would help the children remember to put spaces in between words. Skipping lines on the paper would encourage proper spacing on the paper at large. Using raised line paper would support proper alignment. Finally, using grid paper would address proper sizing of letters and words. *Occupational Therapy for Children* by Case-Smith

139. a. Voluntary hand opening is a requisite skill for active grasp. The ability to actively grasp a toy is not dependent on the other skills. *Hand Function in the Child* by Henderson and Pehoski

140. b. It would be best to first engage the child in a bilateral task that does not require refined movements. Playing catch with a large inflatable beach ball is the only choice that requires gross movements. *Hand Function in the Child* by Henderson and Pehoski

141. a. A notebook under a student's paper will provide additional proprioceptive feedback when writing. *Occupational Therapy for Children* by Case-Smith

142. b. Joint compression will provide the student with the appropriate means of receiving proprioceptive input. The sensory seeking behavior of crashing into the locker, although inappropriate, is a way the child may be seeking proprioceptive input. *Sensory Integration: Theory and Practice* by Bundy

143. a. Contemporary approaches to motor learning support the adaptation and the development of automatic movements by providing tasks that allow the child to develop efficient movement strategies through trial and error. An obstacle course can afford the child with developmental coordination disorder an opportunity to practice the necessary cognitive and motor strategies essential for developing efficient motor patterns. *Pediatric Occupational Therapy and Early Intervention* by Case-Smith

144. d. Providing firm, steady jaw support externally under the base of the tongue and firm but gentle cheek support may help an infant to latch on, strengthen lip seal, and decrease liquid loss. *Occupational Therapy for Children* by Case-Smith

145. d. This type of repetitive contraction is clonus and it best responds to weight bearing. Warmth can be helpful when assisting someone in decreasing spasticity, but would not be helpful in this situation. Clonus is not a volitional response, so asking someone to "relax" is not helpful. Moving someone while he or she is experiencing clonus could actually increase the clonus movement. *Occupational Therapy Practice Skills for Physical Dysfunction* by Pedretti and Early

146. c. A patient with significant spasticity that limits passive wrist and finger extension needs to have a splint that addresses all joints that are involved. A soft device in the palm of the hand may increase spasticity. The cone has an inhibition effect on flexor muscles because it creates deep tendon pressure on the wrist and finger-flexor insertions at the base of the palm. *Introduction to Splinting* by Coppard and Lohman

147. a. Utilizing adaptive equipment, you would expect that he would be independent with the upper portion of his body but need some if not total physical assistance for the lower half of his body. *Occupational Therapy Practice Skills for Physical Dysfunction* by Pedretti and Early

148. b.   Amyotrophic lateral sclerosis is a degenerative disease without a cure that results in death. Stage 3 is characterized by moderate dependence in self-care ADLs and IADLs along with severe weakness of the arms and legs. At this stage of the disease, conserving energy and quality of life are paramount. *Occupational Therapy Practice Skills for Physical Dysfunction* by Pedretti and Early

149. a.   With a C5 spinal cord injury, a person is unable to perform wrist extension or hand movement so the wrist must be supported and the utensil placed in the pocket of the u-cuff so that it can be brought to the mouth using the biceps. A tenodesis splint will not benefit the patient because there is no wrist extension to activate the splint. He will be unable to feed himself with the u-cuff only or without equipment because of a lack of available movement in the wrist. *Occupational Therapy Practice Skills for Physical Dysfunction* by Pedretti and Early

150. a.   If a patient will need to utilize tenodesis to substitute for finger flexion to grasp the item, they will need some tightness in these tendons. This is developed by maintaining finger flexion, with the wrist fully extended and finger extension with the wrist flexed. This prevents the flexors or extensors to be in full stretch, which would prevent any tightness needed for grasp. *Occupational Therapy Practice Skills for Physical Dysfunction* by Pedretti and Early

151. d.   Splints can help prevent contractures and skin breakdown. Before this patient can use their arms functionally, their ROM must be available. *Occupational Therapy Practice Skills for Physical Dysfunction* by Pedretti and Early

152. b.   Although non-slip rugs are good, color is the primary concern in regards to visual acuity. Notifying neighbors would not be considered an adaptive approach. Driving abilities should be addressed by a driver rehabilitation specialist if the vision specialist feels that there may be difficulties. *Vision, Perception and Cognition* by Zoltan

153. b.   An adaptive approach is appropriate when a patient has obviously not had success with remedial activities as mentioned in (a), (c), and (d). *Vision, Perception and Cognition* by Zoltan

154. d.   Although the patient may have these other deficits, we will need further observation and evaluation to deduce that there are difficulties with attention and sequencing, which are both cognitive abilities. Spatial neglect was not mentioned in the

scenario. *Occupational Therapy Practice Skills for Physical Dysfunction* by Pedretti and Early

155. a. Somatagnosia is the inability to recognize one's parts in relationship to each other. Difficulty with sequencing would be noticed in the order the clothes were donned. Spatial neglect could be seen if the patient did not dress a portion of their body. *Vision, Perception and Cognition* by Zoltan

156. b. When someone is able to complete a skill independently in one setting but not transfer this skill to another setting, the person lacks the ability to generalize that skill. They may have difficulty in the other areas that were mentioned, but the OT was not at the group home to assess the situation and the scenario does not clarify what areas were difficult. *Occupational Therapy Practice Skills for Physical Dysfunction* by Pedretti and Early

157. b. Fatigue is a significant issue with multiple sclerosis and management is key to quality of life. End of life issues would not be appropriate because multiple sclerosis is not a terminal illness. The others would be applicable if the patient was having difficulty in these areas. *Occupational Therapy Practice Skills for Physical Dysfunction* by Pedretti and Early

158. c. This is an example of grading an activity by changing food types and increasing the challenge of the task. The others are examples of adapting the activity. *Occupational Therapy Practice Skills for Physical Dysfunction* by Pedretti and Early

159. a. By providing tactile cues to the left side of the body the patient is working on addressing this side. The other treatment suggestions are adaptive by providing the needed objects on the right side of the body. *Occupational Therapy Practice Skills for Physical Dysfunction* by Pedretti and Early

160. b. Discomfort and damage can occur if the scapula is not gliding with the humerus during movement. Passive ROM can cause damage if the structures are not moving properly. An orthopedic specialist may be beneficial if therapy interventions have not been successful. *Occupational Therapy Practice Skills for Physical Dysfunction* by Pedretti and Early

161. b. At level C5, a person may be able to do self-feeding with mobile arm supports and set-up with adapted utensils. The rotator cuff muscles and biceps are partially innervated and weak. The mobile arm support can assist in providing more proximal stability. Grasp is not possible, so a universal cuff to hold

utensils will be needed. *Willard & Spackman's Occupational Therapy,* 10th ed. by Crepeau, Cohn, and Schell

162. d. Although progressive deterioration of skill deficits cannot be prevented, the appropriate level of cues from the social environment can prevent a faster rate of deterioration. *Willard & Spackman's Occupational Therapy,* 10th ed. by Crepeau, Cohn, and Schell

163. d. At 11 months of age, the hyoid and the larynx are more mobile. The pharynx is also elongated. These structural changes require more control by the infant to push the liquid to the entrance of the esophagus. The pull of gravity in a reclined position can interfere with this control and put the infant at a greater risk of aspiration. On the other hand, the epiglottis and soft palate are in direct proximation until about 4 months of age. During swallowing, the larynx elevates and the epiglottis falls over the trachea to protect it, allowing an infant to safely feed in a reclined position until about 4 months of age. A small oral cavity filled with fatty cheeks is the oral structure that exists at birth. This affords a tight fit to the nipple and helps the infant achieve automatic suction. *Occupational Therapy for Children* by Case-Smith

164. c. You would begin with desensitization activities. The texture of a warm washcloth is easily tolerated by most infants and is useful in improving sensory tolerance. Also, you would consider dietary changes and consultation with a nutritionist is important in this regard. The patient would tolerate food if it is placed on the anterior part of the tongue. Although vibration has its benefits when applied to the lower jaw and around the mouth, proximity to the vestibular receptors is likely to cause vestibular system reactions. *Occupational Therapy for Children* by Case-Smith

165. a. Using a spoon with a built-up handle will compensate for limited grasp. The bolster helps increase arm stability, improves position for feeding, and improves the hand movement patterns during feedings. Using a straw can promote the ability to suck and it allows the client to drink without having to lift the cup. A wider and flatter dish would not help as it would be difficult to scoop food out of it. *Occupational Therapy for Children* by Case-Smith

166. c. Soft crackers, such as graham crackers and butter cookies, encourage chewing and also easily dissolve in the mouth. Soft foods reduce the risk of choking. Well-cooked vegetables without skins also promote chewing when placed between teeth.

Soft white bread is not the right texture to introduce to the child because it has a tendency to form a sticky ball and adhere to the upper palate. Dried fruit and pretzels also cannot be considered because they lack moisture. *Occupational Therapy for Children* by Case-Smith

167. a.   For a child who has respiratory disorders that hamper swallowing, an upright feeding position improves respiration and facilitates the coordination of swallowing. *Occupational Therapy for Children* by Case-Smith

168. b.   Using a spoon to create downward pressure on the center of the tongue while feeding will help to promote a sucking pattern and foods such as apple slices, pretzels, and French fries will help increase chewing. Seating in a beanbag chair is not the best option for feeding because postural alignment is difficult to control. Applying touch pressure on the cheeks is appropriate only during bottle-feeding. *Occupational Therapy for Children* by Case-Smith

169. c.   Liquids that have a thicker consistency, such as thick cream soups and thick fruit juices, will be easier to control. Because the child has significant motor problems, thin liquids are contraindicated (water and broths). *Occupational Therapy for Children* by Case-Smith

170. b.   In backward chaining, the OT performs most of the task, and the child performs the last step of a sequence to receive positive reinforcement for completing the task. This method is particularly helpful for children with a low frustration tolerance or poor self-esteem because it gives immediate success. In the restore approach, OTs identify gaps in performance skills and intervene to teach or remediate the underlying problem that is interfering with a child's ADL performance. This approach focuses on the child's deficits in body function and structure. In forward chaining, the child begins with the first step of the task sequence, then the second step, and continues learning steps of the task in a sequential order until he or she can perform all steps in the task. *Occupational Therapy for Children* by Case-Smith

171. c.   For brushing teeth, an enlarged toothbrush handle will make it easier to hold the brush. *Occupational Therapy for Children* by Case-Smith

172. c.   Upper extremity stability and posture are important factors that affect writing. Because the child exhibits poor postural and limb control, he would benefit by postural and limb preparation

activities, such as calisthenics, which would increase muscle tone. The prone position requires forearms to bear the weight and so it increases proximal strength and stability, which would help in better manipulation of writing tools. *Occupational Therapy for Children* by Case-Smith

173. c. A variety of prosthetic devices are available to modify grip patterns. A rubber band sling helps encourages the student to hold the pencil in a slanted and relaxed position. Writing with a wider-barreled pencil helps reduce writing muscle tension and fatigue. *Occupational Therapy for Children* by Case-Smith

174. a. A sensorimotor model of practice is used here to control sensory input through selected activities. Vestibular and auditory input is being provided to help. *Occupational Therapy for Children* by Case-Smith

175. a. Compensatory strategies, such as giving more oral assignments, could be included to help improve grades because the child exhibits a fairly good grasp of content. *Occupational Therapy for Children* by Case-Smith

176. a. A handwriting program should have a structured progression of introducing and teaching letter and number forms. Therefore, it is right to introduce letters with the similar formational features as a family. Writing newly acquired letters and those that have been mastered in a meaningful context is not only more purposeful but also more powerful. *Occupational Therapy for Children* by Case-Smith

177. c. Remedial techniques are those that help in improving or establishing a student's functional skills in a specific area. Using adhesive strips as spacers and providing raised lines as tactile cues for letter placement qualify as remedial measures. These techniques help in written communication. On the other hand, compensatory techniques improve a student's participation in school with adaptations and modifications. Therefore, adding cushions, including more oral activities, and moving a desk away form the window to avoid distractions are all compensatory activities. *Occupational Therapy for Children* by Case-Smith

178. a. The therapist has chosen to use chalk, grease pencils, and other such resistive tools because more pressure is required to write with these than with traditional tools like a pen or pencil. They provide additional proprioceptive input, which helps in better letter formation. *Occupational Therapy for Children* by Case-Smith

179. c. Using a chord keyboard would help hold down more than one key with one hand simultaneously. Chord keyboards have fewer keys, one for each finger, and a couple to be operated by the thumb. *Occupational Therapy for Children* by Case-Smith

180. c. Programs such as a talking word processor will help the child to do writing assignments without getting tired. The talking word processor reads aloud what the student has typed. *Occupational Therapy for Children* by Case-Smith

181. a. Hand-propelled tricycle models are available for children who do not have the ability to pedal with their legs. These can provide mobility outdoors, in hallways, and in corridors. *Occupational Therapy for Children* by Case-Smith

182. b. TOTWalker is a new type of indoor mobility device that would be most suitable. It is designed with minimal hardware in front of the child so he or she can be within arms' reach to access and explore the environment. The TOTWalker allows for a high degree of maneuverability because it has a small turning radius and because placement of the wheel is located near the axis of the child's body. *Occupational Therapy for Children* by Case-Smith

183. b. Wheel locks help with braking, providing stability during transfers. Low seat height is especially important for younger children during transfers and for getting under surfaces like tables. Foot rests will support a child's feet and may act as a step during transfer. If a chair is fitted with these features, it would help considerably. *Occupational Therapy for Children* by Case-Smith

184. c. The infant should feed orally for a few minutes or until cues suggest stress and fatigue. The remainder of the feeding could be given by NGT. When the infant is showing feeding readiness cues, more frequent feeds of shorter durations can occur to avoid prolonged sessions that would tire the infant and decrease feeding safety. This approach would encourage oral feeding and not compromise on nutrition so feeding only by NGT can be avoided. *Occupational Therapy for Children* by Case-Smith

185. c. Hippotherapy is a structured activity that the child participates in, and intentional learning occurs. Playing in the playground and in the sandbox or mother–infant playgroups exemplify unintentional learning through an unstructured activity. *Occupational Therapy for Children* by Case-Smith

186. a. To hammer the nail, the child has to hit the nail every time and it would require use of visual and motor skills. Rotating

small objects in the hand using in-hand manipulation involves tactile perception and isolated finger movement; movement is guided by touch rather than vision. Finger painting is also guided by touch and involves sensory exploration more than eye-hand coordination. *Occupational Therapy for Children* by Case-Smith

187. d.   Adapted utensils for self-feeding would be beneficial and allow for independence. A pressure garment would help a patient with burn injuries to prevent hypertrophic scarring. A patient with juvenile rheumatoid arthritis would need splints. *Occupational Therapy for Children* by Case-Smith

188. c.   Many patients report that they engage in binging behaviors when under stress. Occupational therapy can provide programs in stress management to deal with these issues. Expressive arts can also be helpful, because they are less structured than craft kits.

189. b.   It is important to acknowledge the patient's feelings (and not dismiss or judge him) and then help him understand that your professional role must be maintained. *Mental Health Concepts and Techniques for the Occupational Therapy Assistant* by Early

190. d.   Engaging in deep breathing and relaxation exercises can help her to build skills that she can continue to use. The other activities might serve to increase her anxiety level. *Mental Health Concepts and Techniques for the Occupational Therapy Assistant* by Early

191. a.   The MOHO sees the person as a system, made up of volition, habituation, performance skills, and influenced by the environment. There are a variety of tools available based on this approach that can help a client to better understand their skill capabilities and empower them to rebuild habits and roles that will assist in adjusting to the many changes in life. The other approaches do not take into consideration changing life roles, interests, or volition. *Mental Health Concepts and Techniques for the Occupational Therapy Assistant* by Early and *Group Dynamics in Occupational Therapy* by Cole

192. c.   An assumption of the Cognitive Disabilities Frame of Reference is that limitations in routine task behavior are the result of a physical or chemical dysfunction in the brain. Therefore, emphasis in this approach is placed on the value of assessment and environmental adaptation to positively impact functional performance. *Group Dynamics in Occupational Therapy* by Cole

193. b. Emphasis in this framework is on assessment and management. Dysfunction is caused by a chemical or physical dysfunction in the brain, and it is believed that adapting the environment is the main way to enhance task performance. *Group Dynamics in Occupational Therapy* by Cole

194. b. Psychoanalytic theory emphasizes that behavior is a result of unconscious conflicts and issues that remain unresolved for the individual. The person may display resistance to facing these issues and develop defense mechanisms to ward off anxiety and preserve the ego. Faulty learning's impact on psychopathology is an assumption of a behavioral approach. Physical or chemical dysfunction in the brain and environmental adaptation are associated with the cognitive disabilities approach. *Group Dynamics in Occupational Therapy* by Cole

195. c. Directive groups are particularly beneficial for lower functioning patient groups. They provide predictability and structure and encourage involvement of all members. *Directive Groups* and *Group Dynamics in Occupational Therapy* by Cole

196. b. These techniques use a combination of behavioral and cognitive approaches to assist the patient to build tolerance to anxiety-producing situations. *Psychosocial Occupational Therapy: A Clinical Practice* by Cara and MacRae

197. a. If the behavior is reinforced every single time that it is demonstrated, it is considered continuous reinforcement. *Mental Health Concepts and Techniques for the Occupational Therapy Assistant* by Early and *Group Dynamics in Occupational Therapy* by Cole

198. b. All but the pottery clay are structured activities that limit self-expression. In a psychoanalytical approach you want to encourage self-expression. *Psychosocial Occupational Therapy: A Clinical Practice* by Cara and MacRae and *Group Dynamics in Occupational Therapy* by Cole

199. a. Therapy that addresses sensory issues can impact underlying social and behavioral skills. Training in self-management skills can support ADL performance. *Psychosocial Occupational Therapy: A Clinical Practice* by Cara and MacRae and *DSM-IV-TR*

200. b. The ADL practice will help to re-establish habits of successful self-care performance, and the expressive arts will allow for creative expression of feelings. The other activities are likely to be too threatening and overwhelming to him at this time.

Psychosocial Occupational Therapy: A Clinical Practice by Cara and MacRae

201. c. Reminiscence groups allow for life review to enhance self-integrity and life satisfaction. They can also support re-establishment of normal social functioning. *Group Dynamics in Occupational Therapy* by Cole

202. a. The primary focus at this point should be on creating ways to support occupational functioning. Making a memory book will give the client a useful tool. *Group Dynamics in Occupational Therapy* by Cole

203. b. Even though crafts provide the concrete structure needed by such clients, leatherwork requires an extend attention to task. Psychoeducational and self-esteem building groups require a great deal of processing capacity. Therefore, a group about current events, using a structured directive approach, is the best choice. *Group Dynamics in Occupational Therapy* by Cole

204. d. Cooking, grooming, and work evaluation groups require a higher level of organization. *Psychosocial Occupational Therapy: A Holistic Approach* by Stein and Cutler

205. c. Alzheimer's patients often have difficulty with change. The family members can contribute information about what items are valuable and should be retained and can also assist the client in gradually changing in the environment to reduce stress and allow time to adjust. *Mental Health Concepts and Techniques for the Occupational Therapy Assistant* by Early

206. b. Unless the patient is already physically acting out and creating a safety issue, the patient should be offered the opportunity to leave the group of their own accord, with the responsibility to meet with you later. Using a "show of force" by calling security or making demands of their behavior may only serve to escalate the situation. Should the patient begin to physically act out, then other patients should be removed for their safety and at least two staff should be present when the patient is confronted. *Mental Health Concepts and Techniques for the Occupational Therapy Assistant* by Early and *Psychosocial Occupational Therapy: A Clinical Practice* by Cara and MacRae

207. c. A predominant issue for many of these children is their difficulty in socializing effectively because of their impulsive behavior. Social skills groups can be designed to help them recognize the impact that their behavior has on others

around them and help them to develop such skills in being patient and taking turns. *Psychopathology and Function* by Bonder

208. a. The primary concern of psychosocial rehabilitation is the social aspect of mental illness, not the medical one. Consultation with a psychiatrist may be available through such programs, but it is not an essential service. *Mental Health Concepts and Techniques for the Occupational Therapy Assistant* by Early

209. d. A patient is prescribed fluidotherapy for 20 minutes, then works on buttoning shirt. According to AOTA, OTs should use physical agents' modalities as adjunctive methods to treatment or in preparation for purposeful activity or occupation. *AOTA Physical Agent Modalities: Official Documents*

210. a. Prognosis is determined when the OT considers the severity of the patient's functional limitations and impairments and predicts the possible level of expected improvement or outcome. *Writing Soap Notes* by Kettenbach

211. b. A classic sign of radial nerve compression is wrist drop. If held in this position for an extended period of time, this can lead to overstretching of the forearm extensors muscles and tightness of the forearm flexors. A custom-based dynamic splint with an outrigger that serves to hold the fingers in extension and prevents wrist drop is usually the first step in therapy. This type splint also increase the likelihood of functional hand use. *Hand and Upper Extremity Rehabilitation: A Practical Guide* by Burke, Higgins, McClinton, Saunders, and Valdata

212. a. To decrease the symptoms of thoracic outlet syndrome, which are pain and paresthesias in the neck, shoulder, and arm of the affected extremity, sidelying on the unaffected side with a pillow under the cervical region is the most advantageous position. *Hand and Upper Extremity Rehabilitation: A Practical Guide* by Burke, Higgins, McClinton, Saunders, and Valdata

213. d. An update on the patient's cognitive performance is essential in identifying the performance deficits of someone with a diagnosis of Alzheimer's. *Psychosocial Occupational Therapy: A Clinical Practice* by Cara and MacRae

214. c. An individual with decreased strength, particularly in the lower extremity, would benefit from the use of a sliding board for transfers. *Occupational Therapy Practice Skills for Physical Dysfunction* by Pedretti and Early

215. d. Weighted items, such as heavy pots and pans, will provide more stability for someone who has issues of incoordination. *Occupational Therapy Practice Skills for Physical Dysfunction* by Pedretti and Early

216. a. When performing tasks, particularly to the lower extremity, the client should support the trunk with one extremity while performing tasks with the opposite extremity. *Occupational Therapy for Physical Dysfunction* by Trombly and Radomski

217. b. A person with severe weakness who cannot participate in a transfer should be moved using a dependent transfer. Using a one-person technique, the OT stands in front of the person and places them in a forward flexed position with the chest lying on the thighs. This technique enables greater control over the movement or transfer of the individual. Other methods include a two-person transfer or using a hydraulic or powered lift. *Occupational Therapy for Physical Dysfunction* by Trombly and Radomski

218. b. Principles of compensation support that, when dealing with chronic pain, the OT should reinforce proper body mechanics and pacing of physical tasks. *Occupational Therapy for Physical Dysfunction* by Trombly and Radomski

219. c. Work simplification principles suggest that when fatigue is an issue, work methods should focus on efficiency, such as organizing work areas and storing frequently used items in easily accessible areas. *Occupational Therapy for Physical Dysfunction* by Trombly and Radomski

220. d. To compensate for a progressive condition that has cognitive limitations, such as dementia, use visual and auditory aids to enhance memory and organization. Also, encourage carrying out tasks in familiar environments like the home or various rooms within the house. *Occupational Therapy for Physical Dysfunction* by Trombly and Radomski

221. b. Lapboards are often indicated for persons with poor trunk control and for those who require variability of upper extremity motion. Lapboards can also help to stabilize the upper body and increase the ability to use the proximal extremities. *Occupational Therapy for Physical Dysfunction* by Trombly and Radomski

222. b. Weight cuffs on wrist may help some patients to gain stability and accuracy while performing grooming tasks. *Occupational Therapy for Physical Dysfunction* by Trombly and Radomski

223. a. Persons with a traumatic brain injury may be prone to periods of agitation. When behavior indicating agitation is noted, one strategy is to change the activity or move to a different environment. *Occupational Therapy for Physical Dysfunction* by Trombly and Radomski

224. b. The term "soft end field" is a spongy quality at end range of a joint contracture. It usually indicates that the joint has the potential to remodel. A low load, long duration stretch may yield the best results. *Occupational Therapy for Physical Dysfunction* by Trombly and Radomski

225. c. Active and active assistive ROM is commonly used during periods when joints are inflamed. Using passive stretching during this period can reduce tensile strength and increase inflammation. *Occupational Therapy for Physical Dysfunction* by Trombly and Radomski

226. a. A stress management technique such as visualization helps persons to mentally transport out of stressful anxiety-provoking situations that may be created with episodes of shortness of breath. *Occupational Therapy for Physical Dysfunction* by Trombly and Radomski

227. c. For problems with oral hyposensitivity, the OT should place bolus or flavorful foods in the more sensitive areas of the mouth to stimulate sensation. *Occupational Therapy for Physical Dysfunction* by Trombly and Radomski

228. a. The best recommendation is to assess work areas for the appropriateness of furnishing and accessories. *Occupational Therapy Practice Skills for Physical Dysfunction* by Pedretti and Early

229. b. Persons with visual acuity tend to have problems with low contrast and illumination. Activities focused on increasing the contrast of fore and backgrounds, using large print, bright bold colors, and increased lighting are useful. *Quick Reference Guide to Occupational Therapy* by Reed

230. a. When a person has muscle weakness too great to resist gravity, he or she should be placed in a position of function to minimize edema, minimize the chance of developing deformities, and maintain ROM. *Occupational Therapy Practice Skills for Physical Dysfunction* by Pedretti and Early

231. b. Several stages of sensory reeducation should be addressed following a peripheral nerve injury including object recognition,

object manipulation of various sizes and shapes, control of prehension, and maintenance of prehension force while transporting items. *Occupational Therapy for Physical Dysfunction* by Trombly and Radomski

232. a. Compensatory techniques are necessary when an individual has diminished protective or lacks sensation. The goal of therapy is to avoid injury by teaching the necessary precautions and techniques to avoid tissue damage. *Occupational Therapy for Physical Dysfunction* by Trombly and Radomski

233. c. Desensitization usually involves an area of hypersensitivity. A program of desensitization includes a program of applying different textures and media to a hypersensitive part of the body ranging from soft to coarse. *Occupational Therapy for Physical Dysfunction* by Trombly and Radomski

234. a. Therapeutic exercise should be used as adjunctive therapy or in preparation for functional and purposeful occupational therapy interventions. *Occupational Therapy Practice Skills for Physical Dysfunction* by Pedretti and Early

235. b. Principles of joint protection encourage the use of stronger larger joints to handle greater forces and loads. For example, using the hips and knees to lift or pushing item instead of carrying. *Occupational Therapy for Physical Dysfunction* by Trombly and Radomski

236. b. Apply stimuli using light-moving stroke to the affected area. For hypersensitivity, the first phrase of sensory re-education should consist of using enough pressure to perceive the stimulus but not enough to cause discomfort or pain. *Occupational Therapy for Physical Dysfunction* by Trombly and Radomski

237. b. The patient must be supervised during meals. Supervision requires that a family member or caregiver be present during the activity and assist if required. *Occupational Therapy Practice Skills for Physical Dysfunction* by Pedretti and Early

238. c. Compression, such as with Coban, Isotoner glove, and/or silicone gel pads, helps to soften scar tissue and promote maturation. *Occupational Therapy for Physical Dysfunction* by Trombly and Radomski

239. b. Patients with pulmonary involvement often have limited ability to perform ADLs because of dyspnea. The therapist should note the client's breathing patterns during the activity. Breathing

that becomes shallow and fast indicates a need to reduce or stop the activity. *Occupational Therapy for Physical Dysfunction* by Trombly and Radomski

240. a. Compensatory techniques are used when an individual is not expected to regain or progress with skills or movement. Compensatory methods mean the OT is providing an equivalent solution to achieve a particular skill. In this case, learning to type on a computer would be a compensatory technique for one who has difficulty writing. *Occupational Therapy Practice Skills for Physical Dysfunction* by Pedretti and Early

241. c. Preprosthetic training focuses on promoting readiness for the permanent prosthesis including promoting skin healing, conditioning, preventing contractures, controlling edema, and providing desensitization to the residual limb. *Quick Reference to Occupational Therapy* by Reed

242. d. Interventions for musculoskeletal injuries and conditions, such as tendonitis, fractures, overuse syndromes, and nerve compression injuries, are based on the biomechanical model. The primary goal is improving function by addressing neuromuscular client factors, such as inflammation, edema, motion, strength, endurance, and proprioception. *Quick Reference to Occupational Therapy* by Reed

243. b. Orthostatic hypotension occurs when there is a sudden change in position (usually supine to sit, or sit to stand). A sudden drop in blood pressure is experienced, characterized by dizziness; in severe cases, the individual may lose consciousness. *Quick Reference to Occupational Therapy* by Reed

244. a. A non-skid mat or antislide material is useful in stabilizing dishes so that the individual can scoop and eat independently. *Quick Reference to Occupational Therapy* by Reed

245. c. The OT should encourage weight bearing. Weight bearing through heavy joint compression facilitates co-contraction of the muscles. Placing a person in a quadruped position or leaning on both arms on a table and lifting one limb off the surface produces weight bearing that can improve hypotonia. *Occupational Therapy for Physical Dysfunction* by Trombly and Radomski

246. d. Instructions to reposition, such as chair push ups, side leans, or forward leans, may be used to provide pressure relief and should

be done every 15–30 minutes for individuals who are confined to wheelchairs. Additionally, the individual should be aware of how to examine the body for bruises, redness, and other signs of skin breakdown. *Occupational Therapy for Physical Dysfunction* by Trombly and Radomski

247. c. The copper tooling forms provide tactile input to cue the patient to the boundaries of the picture. The other tasks would be less likely to provide a successful outcome for the patient. *Mental Health Concepts and Techniques for the Occupational Therapy Assistant* by Early

248. d. This response encourages the client to self-evaluate and realistically determine (for himself) if the activity is a good fit. Response (d) avoids the judgmental flavor of the other responses and empowers the patient in skill building. *Mental Health Concepts and Techniques for the Occupational Therapy Assistant* by Early

249. d. This is the most measurable goal focused on the patient's current needs. *Mental Health Concepts and Techniques for the Occupational Therapy Assistant* by Early

250. a. Occupations must be motivating to the patient in order to have the best therapeutic outcome. It is important to learn what interests the client and what will motivate the person to engage in treatment. *Mental Health Concepts and Techniques for the Occupational Therapy Assistant* by Early

251. b. This is an exerci se in planning ahead, which is often a part of a wellness and prevention program. *Mental Health Concepts and Techniques for Occupational Therapy Assistant* by Early

252. a. Wedging clay would allow a way to vent the physical portion of anger in a productive versus destructive way (that the other activities do not) and eventually allow the client to be able to talk more about his feelings. *Mental Health Concepts and Techniques for the Occupational Therapy Assistant* by Early

253. c. Teaching the patient relaxation exercises can help the patient to learn to focus their energy and attention towards healthful activity. *Mental Health Concepts and Techniques for the Occupational Therapy Assistant* by Early

254. a. Giving the patient a written schedule to follow can increase their independence. *Mental Health Concepts and Techniques for the Occupational Therapy Assistant* by Early

255. c. Job hunting on the patient's own has already been unsuccessful and the patient does not need an excessive amount of structure. Too much independence is a set-up for more failure. Using a job coach to help cue them to tasks might provide the needed support and still allow the patient to demonstrate his skills and build self-esteem. *Occupational Therapy in Community-Based Practice Settings* by Scaffa

256. a. Biofeedback is the process of using physical and auditory cues to allow the client to gain control of heart rate and muscle tension. *Psychopathology and Function* by Bonder

257. a. These treatments remain controversial but have helped many patients with depression to function more effectively in normal daily occupations. *Conditions in Occupational Therapy: Effect on Occupational Performance* by Hansen

258. c. Occupational therapy intervention with chronic pain patients involves assessment of their occupational functioning and treatment that empowers them to take control over their lives. *Conditions in Occupational Therapy: Effect on Occupational Performance* by Hansen

259. b. As a holistic practice, occupational therapy provides a wide range of evaluation and treatment services that are designed to meet the patient's current needs. *Conditions in Occupational Therapy: Effect on Occupational Performance* by Hansen

260. d. Examples of compensatory strategies for handwriting difficulties include keyboarding, word prediction, reducing the amount of written work required, allowing oral responses, speech recognition, spell checker, and allowing manuscript rather than cursive writing. *Occupational Therapy for Children* by Case-Smith

261. a. The OT joins the teacher in assisting individual students to complete planned curriculum activities in the classroom. In an integrated therapy model, the practitioner provides intervention in the child's natural environment (e.g., within the classroom, on the playground, in the cafeteria, or on and off the school bus) emphasizing nonintrusive methods. *Occupational Therapy for Children* by Case-Smith

262. a. Integrated therapy allows the OT to provide services in the natural environment. *Occupational Therapy for Children* by Case-Smith

263. d. Proprioceptive sensation about muscle and joint position may result from resistive movement. *Sensory Integration Theory and Practice* by Bundy

264. b. An activity is graded to provide a "just right" challenge when the child is motivated to perform the task, which requires him or her to work while supporting the child's success. *Occupational Therapy for Children* by Case-Smith

265. d. Typical response to a seizure includes timing the event, remaining calm, protecting the child, checking for need of further emergency care after the seizure has concluded, and remaining with the child. *Occupational Therapy for Children* by Case-Smith

266. d. Consultation in an educational setting may include a variety of professionals. Strategies may be aimed at providing an alternative perspective, increasing the student's abilities, or adapting tasks, environments, or routines. *Occupational Therapy for Children* by Case-Smith

267. d. Transition services are those activities that are provided based upon IDEA 2004 to allow disabled students to transition from high school into the community, work, or additional education, whether higher education or technical/vocational training. *OT Services for Children and Youth Under the IDEA* by AOTA

268. a. The Wilbarger approach is an individualized program to treat sensory defensiveness that includes caregiver education, a sensory diet, and possibly deep pressure and proprioceptive input. *Sensory Integration Theory and Practice* by Bundy

269. b. Examples of in-hand manipulation skills include moving small items into the palm of the hand, moving small items from the palm to fingertips, shifting items through hand, and the rotation of small objects between the thumb and index finger. *Occupational Therapy for Children* by Case-Smith

270. a. Using a contrasting background as well as increasing the time visual attention is required would be more appropriate to focus on visual attention deficits. Identifying a removed object and the concentration game would address visual memory. *Occupational Therapy for Children* by Case-Smith

271. d. Pencil grips and altered surfaces are adaptive equipment for handwriting. Hand weights would be a sensorimotor strategy, and Handwriting Without Tears is a handwriting curriculum and intervention program. *Occupational Therapy for Children* by Case-Smith

CHAPTER 7

Questions for Administration and Service Management

Administration refers to managing processes, organizational structure, and nonhuman and human resources to facilitate best practice and delivery of service. Administration takes into account regulations, policies, and procedures that govern the operation of the healthcare organizations and the workplace. In service management, each healthcare practice environment has characteristics that are unique, and occupational therapists (OTs) must provide services within the parameters of that setting. It encompasses being familiar with and adhering to processes related to reimbursement, documentation, consultation, and other areas that distinguish one setting from another.

Both administration and service management are closely linked and work in unison as quality services are delivered to the consumer.

1. The occupational therapy rehabilitation department is conducting outcome studies. Which of the following outcome statements reflects the appropriate way to report the comparison of the consultative and direct models of intervention?
   a. The group receiving consultative intervention achieved a higher number of goals.
   b. The group receiving direct intervention achieved a higher number of goals.
   c. The number of goals achieved was statistically the same when using consultation versus direct intervention.
   d. The goals of both the consultative and direct intervention models were the same.

2. An occupational therapy assistant (OTA) is working with a patient in a community transitional program. The patient is near discharge and needs to have an intervention review. The OT should direct the OTA to:
    a. Select the evaluation methods and measures
    b. Interpret and analyze the assessment data
    c. Complete the interest checklist with the patient
    d. Develop the goals and treatment plan

3. An OT comes to work intoxicated and injures a patient. The OT's license is revoked for 3 years. Which agency/entity is responsible for this disciplinary action?
    a. The American Occupational Therapy Association (AOTA) Commission on Standards and Ethics (SEC)
    b. The Disciplinary Action Committee of the National Board of Certification for Occupational Therapy (NBCOT)
    c. The National Practitioner Data Bank
    d. The State Occupational Therapy Regulatory Board

4. When reviewing license renewals, the occupational therapy director realizes that one OT does not have a current license in the state. Further investigation reveals that the individual never passed the NBCOT certification examination and is not a member of AOTA. The occupational therapy director immediately notifies all pertinent departments/agencies. Which department/agency has NO jurisdiction over this practitioner?
    a. AOTA
    b. Human Resources department
    c. NBCOT
    d. State Regulatory Board

5. An employee in the occupational therapy department repeatedly makes derogatory remarks about a foreign-born therapist. These remarks are made in front of other staff and patients. Which agency is the MOST appropriate choice to report the employee's behavior?
    a. AOTA's Commission on Standards and Ethics (AOTA-SEC)
    b. Equal Employment Opportunity Commission (EEOC)
    c. NBCOT
    d. American Occupational Therapy Foundation (AOTF)

6. Which is NOT a function of NBCOT?
    a. Establishing standards of certification for OT practitioners
    b. Protecting the public from incompetent practitioners
    c. Promoting the growth of the profession of occupational therapy
    d. Granting certificates in recognition of entry-level competence

7. Which statement about NBCOT is NOT true?
   a. The NBCOT certification exam is the same in all 50 states, U.S. territories, and foreign countries where it is given.
   b. Recertification from NBCOT is required in order to use the initials OTR or OTA.
   c. NBCOT is a subsidiary of AOTA.
   d. NBCOT can take disciplinary action against incompetent or unethical OT practitioners or exam candidates.

8. The school-based OT suspected that children with slow handwriting speed would score lower on perceptual motor tests than children with average handwriting speed. The OT reviewed the literature and found a study claiming a correlation between the two issues. The authors reported $P < .05$. The OT found this article to support the theory, because:
   a. <5% of the participants showed a correlation between handwriting speed and perceptual motor skills.
   b. <5% of the participants did not show a correlation between handwriting speed and perceptual motor skills.
   c. <5% probability exists that findings occurred by chance.
   d. <5% of results had to be discarded as inaccurate or unreliable.

9. An OT went to a workshop and learned a new treatment for people with Parkinson's disease. The OT wants to determine if the technique is more beneficial than what is currently being done in the clinic. Using the principles of evidence-based practice (EBP), what is the FIRST step for this OT?
   a. Formulate a specific question comparing the outcomes of the two different treatment approaches
   b. Do an Internet search on treatment of people with Parkinson's disease
   c. Randomly assign clients to one of two treatment groups
   d. Review the occupational therapy textbooks at the local university

10. An OT is trying to determine whether playing music during therapy affects ADL performance. Comparing functional independence measure scores after treatments with and without the music, BEST indicates what aspect of the treatment:
    a. Effectiveness of the treatment
    b. Efficiency of the treatment
    c. Reliability of the treatment
    d. Validity of the treatment

11. Which is MOST likely to be found in quantitative research?
    a. Lengthy, descriptive, narrative text
    b. Open-ended interviewing
    c. Small sample chosen according to goals of the study
    d. Standardized tests and scales

12. An OT is dating a client in the work hardening program. When the client's case manager asks if the patient is ready to return to work, the OT states that additional time in therapy is needed. Which principle of the Code of Ethics has the OT violated?
    a. Autonomy
    b. Beneficence
    c. Fidelity
    d. Nonmaleficence

13. An OTA refuses to teach hemi dressing techniques to a home health client after learning that the client is homosexual. Which principle of the AOTA Code of Ethics has the OTA violated?
    a. Beneficence
    b. Confidentiality
    c. Duties
    d. Veracity

14. The administrator at a hospital wants to start a lymphedema treatment program before a competitor hospital's program opens in 6 months. The occupational therapy director knows that the outpatient therapist has no training in lymphedema treatment but agrees to begin marketing and offering the services immediately. Which principle of the AOTA Code of Ethics has the occupational therapy director violated?
    a. Beneficence
    b. Duties
    c. Fidelity
    d. Justice

15. An OTA called in sick for a week. The supervisor expresses concern to the new department manager and reports that 2 years ago this individual needed a 3-month leave of absence for treatment of severe depression. Which principle of the AOTA Code of Ethics has the occupational therapy supervisor violated?
    a. Autonomy
    b. Fidelity
    c. Nonmaleficence
    d. Veracity

16. An OTA in a long-term care facility forgot to renew the OTA license and informed the facility administrator. The administrator told the OTA that getting the license renewed wasn't necessary because the OTA had current certification from NBCOT. Although the OTA had always renewed the license at a previous job, the OTA did not do it this time. Which principle of the AOTA Code of Ethics did the OTA violate?
    a. Duties

    b. Justice

    c. Nonmaleficence

    d. Veracity

17. An OT walks into a patient's room and finds the patient lying on the floor next to the bed. The OT has been previously reprimanded for forgetting to put the bed rails up after treatment. After checking to be sure the patient has no broken bones and is not in severe pain, the therapist helps the patient back into bed, then leaves the room without reporting the incident. Which terms BEST describe the OT's conduct?

    a. Legal and ethical

    b. Legal but unethical

    c. Ethical but illegal

    d. Illegal and unethical

18. The principle of beneficence is BEST described as:

    a. A healthcare practitioner is required to act as other healthcare professionals would act in similar situations

    b. A healthcare practitioner should act in ways that do not cause harm or injury to others

    c. A healthcare practitioner is required to present choices so that individuals are able to select the best choice for treatment

    d. A healthcare practitioner should act in ways to promote the welfare of other people

19. An occupational therapy manager is asked to prepare a report of revenue for the cardiac program. The manager budget would MOST likely show:

    a. Income

    b. Operating costs

    c. Capital equipment expenses

    d. Direct expenses

20. An occupational therapy manager must prepare a capital budget to request a piece of equipment. The item that would MOST likely be listed in this budget is:

    a. Dynamometer

    b. Fluido-therapy machine

    c. An office chair

    d. Splinting materials

21. The occupational therapy department has had three recent resignations and is short-staffed. The Rehab Director reassigns the psychiatric OT to outpatient clinic 2 days per week. A patient comes in with orders for a specific technique related to lymphedema management, and the OT asks that the patient be reassigned

because the OT has never had any training in this area. Despite the director's insistence, the OT requests that someone with expertise treat the patient. Which core value and attitude of occupational therapy is BEST exemplified by this therapist's action?
a. Altruism
b. Justice
c. Prudence
d. Truth

22. The new OTA in a large university medical center has 3 years experience in a small community outpatient clinic that served adults only. Which BEST describes the appropriate level of supervision that the OT should provide?
a. Close supervision on all units
b. Close supervision in special units such as intensive care and routine supervision on other units
c. Routine supervision on all units
d. Routine supervision for adult patients and close supervision for pediatric patients

23. An OTA with 8 years of experience transfers from the substance abuse unit to the orthopedic team. After saying "you remember hip precautions," the supervisor sends the OTA to treat a patient who underwent a total hip arthroplasty 3 days ago. While practicing dressing, the patient leans forward to do shoe tying and has immediate pain in the operative hip. Two days later the patient has to undergo additional surgery. Liability in this case is the primary responsibility of:
a. The OTA
b. The OT
c. Both the OTA and the OT
d. The physician

24. Which statement is NOT true regarding Medicare Home Health regulations?
a. A client must need skilled nursing, physical therapy, and/ or speech-language pathology services before receiving occupational therapy services.
b. Occupational therapy must discharge the client from services when all other services are ended.
c. Most home healthcare services are provided under Part A.
d. Home health agencies are paid a single rate for each 60 days of services, with higher rates being possible if a specific level of therapy is provided.

25. Reimbursement rates vary according to the type of reimbursement system. Which statement is true regarding reimbursement?
a. There is an incentive for physicians to limit costs in a *fee-for-service* system.

    b. Medicaid is a *prospective* system.

    c. *Capitation* rates vary according to how many patients were treated that month.

    d. A *prospective* system covers all costs for a specific illness for a specified period of time.

26. As healthcare costs escalate, healthcare providers and third-party payers work to develop systems to contain costs. The various payment models shift the risk between the provider and the payer. Which statement is NOT true?

    a. In a *fee-for-service* system the payer has the risk because it must pay all covered costs.

    b. In *capitation* the payer has the risk because many enrollees might receive service in the same month.

    c. In a *prospective* system the provider has the risk because costs might exceed payment.

    d. In a *fee-for-service* system the payer can cut costs by negotiating rates.

27. A patient received several rehab therapies including occupational therapy five times per week for 6 weeks following a fall with resultant elbow and hip fracture and surgical repair. In which setting was the patient MOST likely seen for this length of stay?

    a. Inpatient acute

    b. Inpatient rehab

    c. Skilled nursing facility

    d. Home health

28. When completing the budget variance each month, the occupational therapy director must explain why actual expenses were greater or lower than budgeted expenses. Which of the following items in the variance report is an operating (or indirect) expense, as opposed to a direct expense?

    a. Salary for therapists

    b. Phone bill

    c. Medical/surgical supplies (splinting material)

    d. Storeroom supplies (lymphedema bandages and electrodes)

29. The occupational therapy director is preparing the operating and capital budget for next fiscal year. There are several items needed for the occupational therapy department. Which of these items is NOT a capital expense?

    a. Fluidotherapy machine to replace old one ($4500)

    b. Two new pediatric assessment kits ($400 each)

    c. Large splint pan ($750)

    d. Refrigerator for ADL kitchen ($900)

30. The new pediatric clinic had net revenue of $400,000 last year and expenses of $370,000. What was the profit margin for the clinic?
    a. 5%
    b. 7.5%
    c. 12%
    d. 25%

31. The inpatient department strives for 75% productivity for all therapy staff. Today the OT worked for 9 hours. The OT attended a 1-hour staff meeting and met with an occupational therapy student for 45 minutes after lunch. How much time can the OT allot to documentation and still meet the productivity goal for the day?
    a. .5 hour
    b. 1 hour
    c. 1.5 hour
    d. 2 hours

32. In order to ensure the quality of occupational therapy education, academic programs must meet the minimum standards established by the:
    a. ACOTE
    b. AOTA
    c. CHEA
    d. U.S. Department of Education

33. A chiropractor advertises occupational therapy services in her office, although neither an OT nor an OTA is employed. To be considered legal, the chiropractor is MOST likely practicing in a state with what form of occupational therapy regulation?
    a. Certification
    b. Licensure
    c. Registration
    d. Title control

34. State regulatory agencies often require occupational therapy practitioners to provide proof of continuing competence when renewing licensure, registration, or certification. What evidence is MOST often used to demonstrate continuing competence?
    a. Certificate of moral character
    b. Continuing education credits
    c. NBCOT certification
    d. Absence of any disciplinary action

35. An OT suspects physical abuse after noticing bruises on the face and back of a child during the treatment session. The appropriate action to take is:
    a. To ask the child questions about the bruises
    b. To confront the parents about the cause for the inflictions

    c. To make a report to the appropriate authorities

    d. To ignore the bruises because proof of suspicion is difficult

36. Which of the following is considered an emerging practice area for occupational therapy?
    a. Hand therapy
    b. Functional capacity evaluations
    c. Ergonomic consulting
    d. School system pediatric

37. A main objective of writing a business plan is to:
    a. Market the business to potential customers
    b. Share critical business information with decision makers
    c. Establish departmental policies and procedures
    d. Grow the business over a specified period of time

38. The occupational therapy supervisor evaluates the staff's performance by comparing the individual's productivity to the department's productivity standard. This is an example of:
    a. Controlling
    b. Budgeting
    c. Staffing
    d. Decision making

39. The hospital administrator is concerned about numerous billing errors in the outpatient rehab department. A new occupational therapy manager has been hired and charged by the hospital administrator to review and correct the billing processes. An initial step to rectify this situation would be to:
    a. Educate the staff to assign proper *International Classification of Diagnoses* (ICD) codes to patients when admitted
    b. Educate the staff to assign proper *Current Procedural Terminology* (CPT) codes to patients when charging for evaluations and treatments
    c. Ensure that the staff is reaching productivity standards by reviewing policies and procedures
    d. Teach the billing clerk how to catch and rectify mistakes in billing that are made by the staff

40. To facilitate effective communication between an occupational therapy supervisor and employee, the supervisor should:
    a. Communicate what is expected of the employee
    b. Express disappointment regarding the employee's behavior
    c. Offer criticism to stimulate discussion
    d. Meet with the employee away from the workplace to facilitate a conversation

41. The following are all examples of advocacy by OTs, except:
    a. Seeking a referral for a client
    b. Writing letters of support for a piece of proposed legislation
    c. Joining a professional association and serving on a political action committee
    d. Attending continuing education sessions to advancing your clinical skills

42. An OT is the new director of a comprehensive rehabilitation facility. As the director, the OT leads a group of OTs, OTAs, physical therapists, physical therapy assistants, speech language pathologists, and therapy aides. Within the first week on the job, the director becomes aware of the fact that therapy aides perform multiple tasks including patient transporting, setting up and cleaning the treatment area, and conducting therapy groups without routine supervision. The director knows that such action is in violation of the state's occupational therapy Practice Act. The BEST course of action by the new director is:
    a. Nothing, because the facility's chief operating officer reported that the facility has operated in this manner for the past 5 years
    b. Review the practice act with your staff and require full compliance with state regulations
    c. Contact the facility's administration and lodge a complaint
    d. Allow the aides to continue with present job duties and require therapists to provide close supervision during therapy groups

43. Which of the following characteristics distinguishes a leader from a manager?
    a. Looks to the future
    b. Focuses on daily operations
    c. Maintains the status quo
    d. Focuses on efficiency

44. An administrator of occupational therapy would design a strategic plan for the purpose of:
    a. Developing new service lines and measuring outcomes
    b. Receiving insurance reimbursement
    c. Providing disciplinary actions
    d. Providing feedback to employees on work performance

45. Medicare Part A is referred to as:
    a. Hospital insurance
    b. Supplementary medical insurance
    c. Federal-state medical insurance
    d. A managed care program

46. An OT observes a peer (co-worker) acting in an unethical manner with a client and reports the individual to the appropriate agency (e.g., state licensure board). This action is an example of:

a. Client advocacy
b. Organization advocacy
c. Healthcare environment advocacy
d. Professional advocacy

47. The director of occupational therapy was approached by the hospital's administration to establish "new and profitable" lines of rehabilitation services. The director has identified hand therapy as a potential service and proceeds to develop a business plan. The FIRST market analysis activity that should be undertaken to initiate the business plan is to:
   a. Clearly identify the potential or existing clients' needs and wants
   b. Persuade the potential referral sources to utilize the proposed service
   c. Create awareness of the service
   d. Increase accessibility to the consumer

48. The owner of a freestanding outpatient rehabilitation clinic decides to perform an organizational assessment using a Strength, Weakness, Opportunity, and Threat (SWOT) Analysis to reevaluate the clinic's effectiveness relative to the patient population, the community, and the healthcare system. The owner finds that reimbursement from workers' compensation insurers has decreased by an average of 7% per year for the last 3 years. Using the SWOT analysis tool, the director determines that this is a:
   a. Strength (internal factor)
   b. Weakness (internal factor)
   c. Opportunity (external factor)
   d. Threat (external factor)

49. The OT director must determine the staffing needs of a new home health department. Twenty-four hours of patient treatment are projected for each day of the week. Each OT's productivity is expected to be 6 hours per day. How many full-time equivalent (FTE) therapists would the occupational therapy director need to hire to complete the work each day?
   a. 2 FTEs
   b. 3 FTEs
   c. 4 FTEs
   d. 5 FTEs

50. The occupational therapy manager plans to hire an aide/technician to work in a large occupational therapy department that provides services in both an inpatient and outpatient setting. This is a newly created position, which requires the manager to develop a written job description. In order to comply with the Americans

with Disabilities Act of 1990 (ADA; Public Law 101–336), the occupational therapy manager must identify:
a. Essential and marginal job functions
b. The type of person suited for the job
c. The policy for hiring employees
d. The department's productivity standard

51. The rehab manager has recently hired an OT with a disability. The manager must make reasonable accommodations as required by the Americans with Disabilities Act of 1990 (ADA; Public Law 101–336). All of the following are examples of reasonable accommodations, except:
a. Medication monitoring
b. Modified work schedules
c. Physical changes to the workstation
d. Adjustment of supervisory methods

52. The executive director of rehabilitation services has asked the occupational therapy department manager to collect data for program evaluation. According to the *OT Practice Framework: Domain and Process*, which one of the following service delivery components provides the BEST data to inform program evaluation?
a. Evaluation
b. Intervention
c. Discharge
d. Outcomes

53. The occupational therapy manager recognizes that limited growth opportunities are the main contributing factor to the recently experienced high turnover rates. In order to recruit and retain qualified staff, the MOST effective strategy for the occupational therapy manager to employ to combat high turnover of employees would be:
a. Involve employees in the work design process and create development opportunities
b. Provide formal mechanisms and encourage employees to express work-related concerns
c. Use market information to determine wage and benefit programs
d. Match employee skills with the job and define job prior to employment

54. The occupational therapy manager recognizes that the department has pay inequities, which has led to several employees' resignation over the past 6 months. In order to achieve equitable pay, the MOST effective strategy for the occupational therapy manager to employ is to:
a. Involve employees in the work design process and create development opportunities

b. Provide formal mechanisms and encourage employees to express work-related concerns

c. Use market information to determine wage and benefit programs

d. Match employee skills with the job and define job prior to employment

55. Several teachers inquire about a child's eligibility to receive occupational therapy services. The OT should educate the teachers that a child is eligible for school-based occupational therapy services when the:

a. Parents demand service

b. Principal determines that occupational therapy is needed

c. Child's ability interferes with the child's educational goals

d. Teacher completes the appropriate paperwork for a referral

56. As life expectancy increases, attention needs to be directed toward services that will be required in the future. In addition to healthcare, education, transportation, and recreation, a community-based priority for occupational therapy practice is:

a. Housing

b. Adult daycare

c. Spirituality

d. Leisure

57. At a skilled nursing facility, a team of rehabilitation professionals has received orders for therapy to assess function, gait, transfers, and bed mobility. In addition to the OT, other member of the professional team should include the:

a. Orthopedic doctor and physical therapy

b. Physical therapy and nursing staff

c. Physical therapy and chaplain

d. Speech therapy and nursing staff

58. A 3-year-old has muscular dystrophy and is often hospitalized. The child has acute exacerbation of asthma. What kind of hospital care would this require?

a. Critical care and periodic hospitalization

b. Intensive care and periodic hospitalization

c. Acute care and periodic hospitalization

d. Special medical care and ambulatory services

59. An 8-year-old child will require ongoing services after being discharged from the hospital rehabilitation unit to home. The most effective way that the OT can facilitate transition is to:

a. Organize a meeting between the school and the rehab team

b. Discuss the need for a referral with the doctor

c. Facilitate a meeting between Medicaid services and the family

d. Provide a list of community occupational therapy practitioners to the family

60. A 6-year-old with cerebral palsy has this service mandated under the Individuals with Disabilities Education Act (IDEA) Part B:
    a. Family training, counseling, and home visits
    b. Limited access to specialized services
    c. Interdisciplinary assessment
    d. Discipline specific education assessment

61. The Rehab Director is interested in expanding occupational therapy services to include a hand rehab clinic. In order to validate the support for such as program, the director should conduct:
    a. A market analysis
    b. An organizational assessment
    c. A promotional campaign
    d. A program evaluation

62. The administrator of an outpatient rehabilitation center files a complaint against a staff OT with the Ethics Commission (EC) for an ethical violation. As a final action by the EC, the individual was given a reprimand. Which scenario represents this disciplinary action?
    a. The individual was suspended from practicing for 3 months.
    b. A letter was sent to the individual identifying the issue and expressing disapproval of the behavior.
    c. The individual was placed on probation and monitored by the administrator for a specified period of time.
    d. The name of the individual and the action committed was published in the state occupational therapy licensure board newsletter.

63. A student on affiliation notices that their supervisor routinely documents treatment units before actually seeing the patient. The student discussed this with the administrator because in the Code of Ethics, this action would violate what principle?
    a. Duty
    b. Altruism
    c. Confidentiality
    d. Veracity

64. The insurance company of a client being seen by the OT requests information on the client's status. The OT should:
    a. Ask the insurance company to put their request in writing before sending the information
    b. Obtain written approval from the client before releasing the information
    c. Tell the client to send the information to the insurance company
    d. Ask the administrator to communicate with the insurance company about the client's status

65. As a result of a complaint, the Ethics Commission agreed on disciplinary action in which licensure to practice was removed for 1 year. This punitive action represents:
    a. Suspension
    b. Censure
    c. Revocation
    d. Reprimand

66. Which scenario represents a Sua Sponte Complaint to the Ethics Commission?
    a. The state licensure board informs the Ethics Commission about disciplinary action taken on individual due to unethical behavior.
    b. An OT complains to the Ethics Commission that their supervisor was unethical with billing practices.
    c. The administrator files a complaint that the OT treated patients of one ethnic group different than other individuals.
    d. The physician sends a letter of complaint stating that the therapist was using inappropriate treatment techniques for a particular group of patients.

67. The OTA asked the OT to explain the term "service competency." The BEST response is to explain that service competency:
    a. Is established when a therapist passes the certification exam
    b. Is achieved when an individual attains a certain number of continuing education units
    c. Means individual competency is gained after years of practice
    d. Occurs when two practitioners performing the same procedure gain the same results

68. What legislation grants parents and students access to and confidentiality of educational records?
    a. IDEA
    b. The Family Educational Rights and Privacy Act
    c. Americans with Disabilities Act
    d. The Social Security Act

69. What Medicare Prospective Payment System (PPS) would an OT employed in a long term care facility to direct therapy and billing procedures?
    a. Resource Utilization Grouping (RUGs)
    b. Diagnostic Related Groups (DRGs)
    c. Case Mix Groups (CMGs)
    d. Resource-Based Relevant Value Scale (RBRVS)

70. A key step in strategic planning and setting up programs and goals in healthcare organizations is to use a Strengths, Weaknesses,

Opportunities, and Threats (SWOT) Analysis. What is the purpose of a SWOT analysis?
   a.   To identify the step to program development
   b.   To examine effects of interval and external environments of the organization
   c.   To address laws governing the operation of the organization
   d.   To examine global and international trends affecting the organization

71.   In the Core Values and Attitude document, the specific core value that emphasizes the importance of valuing the inherent worth and uniqueness of each person is:
   a.   Justice
   b.   Dignity
   c.   Prudence
   d.   Altruism

72.   The term that refers to the process of providing information to individuals to assist them in the decision-making process about their own healthcare is:
   a.   Beneficence
   b.   Fidelity
   c.   Autonomy
   d.   Informed consent

73.   Occupational therapy services are covered under Medicare when:
   a.   Prescribed by a physician and considered reasonable and necessary
   b.   Initiated by an occupational therapist in private practice
   c.   The OT has liability insurance
   d.   Other services such as physical therapy and speech are covered

74.   The hospital administrator presents an in-service to employees about a policy that governs the interchange of healthcare information and financial data, and protects the confidentiality of patients. This policy is the known as the:
   a.   Americans with Disabilities Act (ADA)
   b.   Health Insurance Portability and Accountability Act (HIPAA)
   c.   IDEA
   d.   Family Educational Rights and Privacy Act (FERPA)

75.   An OT has a private practice ergonomics consulting business. The OT has been asked to consult with a local textile plant on ergonomic issues. According to the consultation process, what is the FIRST step the therapist should follow?
   a.   Assessment and communication
   b.   Interactive problem solving
   c.   Evaluation and termination
   d.   Initiation and clarification

76. The director of an adult day care center for individuals with Alzheimer's requests assistance from an occupational therapy consultant to provide information on how to identify the earliest warning signs of deterioration in persons with Alzheimer's so that immediate intervention could be provided. The OT reports that the main problem associated with the early stages of Alzheimer's is:
   a. Memory impairment
   b. Repetitive speech
   c. Incontinence
   d. Mood swings

77. An OT is conducting a research study on the effects of splinting in reducing carpal tunnel syndrome. One group in the study receives the splinting treatment and a second group receives an exercise program. In this type of research the group receiving the exercise program is called the:
   a. Experimental group
   b. Population
   c. Control group
   d. Sampling group

78. In a research proposal, what would the following statement represent? "There is a statistically significant difference in reduced symptoms in persons with carpal tunnel when splinting as compared to using a home exercise program."
   a. Hypothesis
   b. Null hypothesis
   c. Independent variable
   d. Dependent variable

79. An occupational therapy student on fieldwork receives a referral to evaluate a client diagnosed with coronary artery bypass surgery. Identify the sequence the student would follow during the evaluation (according to the *OT Practice Framework*):
   a. Gather significant medical data, create occupational profile, administer assessments, develop problem list, formulate goals, and plan the intervention
   b. Create occupational profile, administer assessments, gather significant medical data, develop problem list, formulate goals, and plan the intervention
   c. Administer assessments, develop problem list, gather significant medical data, formulate goals, and plan the intervention
   d. Create occupational profile, gather significant medical data, administer assessments, develop a problem list, formulate goals, and plan the intervention

80. The occupational therapy practitioner is reviewing the literature to determine the best treatment technique to use with a patient. When evaluating evidence-based research, the level of evidence that is considered to be the strongest is attributed to:
    a. Case studies
    b. Cross-sectional surveys
    c. Cohort studies
    d. Randomized control trials

81. Using a formative program evaluation process, the occupational therapy supervisor must assess the effectiveness of rehab services in an inpatient facility. What type of information would be useful to analyze in a formative program evaluation?
    a. Changes in a specific group of patients' level of assistance at discharge
    b. The level of satisfaction of recipients of a newly implemented program
    c. Feedback on the new billing procedures that was recently implemented
    d. Input on the number of persons completing a program successfully

82. A patient tells the OT how much the services provided have helped in coping with their depression. The patient then offers a gift of appreciation to the therapist. The OT's BEST response is to say:
    a. "I love the gift, but I need to report it to my administrator in order to follow regulations."
    b. "Thank you, that's great. What is it?"
    c. "Just knowing that you appreciate my helped is reward enough. I appreciate the gesture, but I cannot accept the gift."
    d. "Please mail it to my house. I cannot accept the gift on the hospital premises."

83. An OT using the evidence-based practice approach to determine the BEST intervention for treating a complicated diagnosis must first:
    a. Search and sort the evidence
    b. Formulate the question
    c. Conduct a literature search
    d. Appraise the evidence

84. The "stress-vulnerability model" refers to:
    a. The impact that environmental stress can have on the functioning of mentally ill patients in the community, especially those diagnosed with schizophrenia

    b. The stress caused by the lack of governmental funding for mental health services

    c. The vulnerability in our healthcare systems caused by the increasing number of mentally ill patients

    d. The stress on the community caused by mentally ill individuals that have been de-institutionalized

85. Which of the following statements is true?
    a. OTs working in mental health have prescription privileges.
    b. OTs working in mental health are allowed to treat patients without a doctor's order.
    c. OTs working in mental health do not diagnose patients.
    d. OTs working in mental health are now considered "qualified mental health providers" (QMHPs) in all 50 states.

86. In community-based occupational therapy mental health services the primary role of the OT is:
    a. Educator
    b. Clinician or case manager
    c. Job coach
    d. Supervisor

87. Which of the following is a true statement?
    a. OTs practicing in mental health never address the physical needs of their clients.
    b. OTs practicing in mental health are required to have a specialty mental health certification.
    c. OTs only address their patients' psychosocial issues in mental health settings.
    d. OTs practicing in mental health address the holistic needs of their clients.

88. In working with psychiatric patients, it is important to:
    a. Involve their families whenever appropriate and possible
    b. Treat the patient without reviewing their histories to avoid prejudging them
    c. Never trust what their families say about them, because most of them are mentally ill, too
    d. Warn the community that they live in about their mental illness

89. Patients with mental illness:
    a. Are always unpredictable
    b. Are usually out of control
    c. Can frequently benefit from occupational therapy services
    d. Are often too sick to benefit from occupational therapy services

90. A female patient privately shares with the OT that she was sexually abused as a child. The OT should:
   a. Share this information with team members to ensure that the care provided is appropriate
   b. Promise not to share the information because it was communicated privately
   c. Inform others during the group therapy session, so that they will give the patient support
   d. Encourage the patient to disclose this information in group therapy to help others who may have had similar experiences

91. Which of the following is a syndrome that occurs as a result of long-term use of antipsychotic medications?
   a. Tardive dyskinesia
   b. Echolalia
   c. Pica
   d. Tachycardia

92. An OT working at an inpatient rehabilitation unit would need to be familiar with the Medicare prospective payment system that classifies patients into categories based on:
   a. Resource utilization groups (RUGs)
   b. Diagnostic related groups (DRGs)
   c. Case mix groups (CMGs)
   d. Resource-based relative value scale (RBRVS)

93. A quadriplegic patient confesses to the OT that he is concerned about meeting his wife's sexual needs now that he is paralyzed. The BEST response of the OT would be to:
   a. Recommend to the physician that the patient begin taking antidepressants because he is probably depressed
   b. Tell the patient to discuss this issue with his wife and work it out between them
   c. Allow the patient to talk about his concerns, explore options, and offer to refer him to a specialist with expertise on this issue
   d. Refer the patient to a psychologist, because talking about these issues is beyond the scope of occupational therapy practice

94. In a skilled nursing facility, the patient's need for services and the prospective per diem rate are established by a resident assessment tool called the:
   a. Minimum Data Set
   b. Functional Independent Measures
   c. Canadian Occupational Performance Measure
   d. RBRVS

95. An occupational therapist involved with a self-help group for patients with the diagnosis of "panic disorder with agoraphobia" would MOST likely take the role of a:
    a. Consultant
    b. Primary group leader
    c. Case manager
    d. Full group member

96. Individuals diagnosed with "oppositional defiant disorder" in childhood or adolescence are MOST often diagnosed with which of the following conditions when they reach adulthood:
    a. Bipolar disorder
    b. Antisocial personality disorder
    c. Schizophrenia
    d. Borderline personality disorder

97. Which of the following is the BEST example of an IEP present level of performance statement based on a school-based OT's evaluation?
    a. The student requires moderate assistance with toileting and minimal assistance with self-feeding.
    b. The student demonstrates a fine motor skill age equivalent of 36 months on the Peabody Developmental Motor Scales.
    c. The student demonstrates sensory processing differences, including sensory defensiveness.
    d. The student is unable to name or legibly write letters and numbers because of delayed visual motor skills.

98. The following are considered primary services under the Individuals with Disabilities Education Act (IDEA):
    a. Specially designed instruction (special education)
    b. Occupational therapy and speech therapy
    c. Occupational therapy and physical therapy
    d. Transportation and psychological services

99. State and local educational agencies may fund related services through the following resources, except:
    a. Private insurance
    b. State Medicaid agencies
    c. Noneducational public agencies
    d. Direct billing to families

100. Which of the following statements describe the collaborative relationship between the OT and the OTA in a school-based setting?
    a. The OT may assign the OTA to perform all aspects of service.
    b. The OTA is responsible for seeking the supervision required for delegated areas of intervention.

    c. The OTA establishes intervention priorities.

    d. The OT is accountable for implementation of intervention.

101. An IEP team meeting MUST include each of the following except:
   a. A regular education teacher's attendance
   b. A review of the student's strengths
   c. The parents' attendance
   d. A physician's attendance

102. An occupational therapy assistant with 5 years of experience in a mental health setting is being reassigned to work in an orthopedic outpatient rehabilitation center. What level of supervision should the OT provide?
   a. Close
   b. Routine
   c. General
   d. Minimal

103. An occupational therapy assistant works in a skilled nursing facility and is supervised by direct contact every 2 weeks with interim written or verbal communication. When performing the employee's appraisal, the director should document the level of supervision for the assistant as:
   a. Close
   b. Routine
   c. General
   d. Minimal

104. An OT employed for less than a year on an acute care unit has mastered the basis routine and job requirements but continues to need mentoring when working on specialty units such as cardiac critical care. What level of role performance is the OT apparently functioning?
   a. Entry level
   b. Intermediate level
   c. Advance level
   d. Supervisory level

105. An employer requests that the OT makes recommendations about universal design in the new retirement complex. The OT would MOST likely recommend:
   a. Placing labels in Braille to identity the rooms of the housing units
   b. Placing railing and bars in the bathrooms and on stairs or steps
   c. Installing a pool for recreational purposes
   d. Creating walking trails within the residential neighborhood

106. An OT acting in the role of a consultant in a school-based setting would:
    a. Teach a child how to tie their shoes
    b. Hold an educational session for parents on sensory integration during play activities
    c. Assist the teacher in learning techniques to assist children with handwriting
    d. Work on feeding techniques with a child who has cerebral palsy

Answers to Administration and Service Management Questions

1. c. The number of occupational therapy goals when using consultation versus direct intervention did not differ (was essentially the same). In research, comparison of two variables can be stated as statistical differences or similarities. Although consultation is an indirect form of intervention, it appears to be as effective as direct services. *Clinical Research in Occupational Therapy* by Stein and Cutter

2. c. According to the Standards of Practice for Occupational Therapy, an OTA would perform functions such as administering some of the assessments and documenting some of the results. Selecting evaluation methods and measures, interpreting and analyzing assessment data, and developing the goals and treatment plan are functions of the registered OT. *Willard & Spackman's Occupational Therapy* by Neidstadt and Crepeau

3. d. State regulatory boards have the power to discipline practitioners through a variety of sanctions ranging from reprimand to revocation of license, certification, or registration. *The Occupational Therapy Manager* by McCormack, Jaffe, and Goodman-Lavey

4. a. Because membership is voluntary, AOTA has no direct, legal jurisdiction over practitioners who are not members. *Willard & Spackman's Occupational Therapy,* 10th ed. by Crepeau, Cohn, and Schell

5. a. Ethical violations of professional values that have no potential to cause harm are likely of interest to AOTA alone. The OT's actions violate the AOTA core value of equality. The SEC is responsible for reviewing allegations about unethical behavior by AOTA members. *Willard & Spackman's Occupational Therapy,* 10th ed. by Crepeau, Cohn, and Schell

6. c. Promoting the growth of the profession of occupational therapy is the purpose of the American Occupational Therapy Association (AOTA). *The Occupational Therapy Manager* by McCormack, Jaffe, and Goodman-Lavey

7. c. NBCOT is an independent organization, formerly known as AOTCB, which was created by AOTA in 1986. *The Occupational Therapy Manager* by McCormack, Jaffe, and Goodman-Lavey

8. c. p = chance that the findings are the result of an error in the study procedures. Usually p values of 1%, 2%, or 5% are used. *Willard & Spackman's Occupational Therapy,* 10th ed. by Crepeau, Cohn, and Schell

9. a. In EBP, a well-formulated question that includes the problem or patient, the intervention, the comparison intervention, and the outcomes becomes the basis for examining the research literature. *The Occupational Therapy Manager* by McCormack, Jaffe, and Goodman-Lavey

10. a. Comparing outcome measures such as the FIM can provide evidence of effectiveness of a treatment intervention. *The Occupational Therapy Manager* by McCormack, Jaffe, and Goodman-Lavey

11. d. Quantitative research answers questions that require standardized measures. Qualitative methods lend themselves to the study of small groups with research questions that may be broad and evolve throughout the study process. *Willard & Spackman's Occupational Therapy,* 10th ed. by Crepeau, Cohn, and Schell

12. d. Principle 2 of the Code of Ethics (nonmaleficence), states that "occupational therapy practitioners shall avoid relationships or activities that interfere with professional judgment and objectivity." *The Occupational Therapy Manager* by Mormack, Jaffe, and Goodman-Lavey

13. a. Principle 1 (beneficence) states that occupational therapy personnel shall provide services in a fair and equitable manner. They shall recognize and appreciate the cultural components of economics, geography, race, ethnicity, religious and political factors, marital status, sexual orientation, and disability of all recipients of their services. *The Occupational Therapy Manager* by McCormack, Jaffe, and Goodman-Lavey

14. b. Principle 4 (duties) states that occupational therapy practitioners shall protect service recipients by ensuring that duties assumed by or assigned to other occupational therapy personnel match credentials, qualifications, experience, and scope of practice. *The Occupational Therapy Manager* by McCormack, Jaffe, and Goodman-Lavey

15. b. Principle 7 (fidelity) states that occupational therapy personnel shall preserve, respect, and safeguard confidential information about colleagues and staff, unless otherwise mandated by

national, state, or local laws. *The Occupational Therapy Manager* by AOTA Press

16. b. Principle 5 (justice) states that occupational therapy personnel shall familiarize themselves with and seek to understand and abide by applicable Association policies; local, state, and federal laws; and institutional rules. *The Occupational Therapy Manager* by McCormack, Jaffe, and Goodman-Lavey

17. b. The behavior was legal because there was no crime and it brought no harm to the patient. It was unethical because the therapist was more concerned about the therapist's needs than the patient's needs. It also violated the principle of veracity. *Ethics in Rehabilitation* by Kornblau and Starling

18. d. Beneficence refers to actions that benefit others. choice (a) describes the reasonable prudent man theory; choice (b) the principle of nonmaleficence; and (c) the definition of rights. *The Occupational Therapy Manager* by AOTA Press and *Ethics in Rehabilitation* by Kornblau and Starling

19. a. Revenue reflects the amount of real dollars collected or the income. *The Occupational Therapy Manager* by McCormack, Jaffe, and Goodman-Lavey

20. b. A capital budget usually consists of a request for large, high-cost equipment (typically $1,000 or more) that has an expected useful life of 3–5 years. When requesting capital equipment, managers usually include a written justification for the equipment to support the expense. *The Occupational Therapy Manager* by McCormack, Jaffe, and Goodman-Lavey

21. d. According to the Core Values and Attitudes of Occupational Therapy Practice, truth requires that practitioners be faithful to facts and reality and are accountable, honest, and accurate in their actions. This includes the accurate representation of one's knowledge and skills. *Effective Documentation for Occupational Therapy* by AOTA and *Willard & Spackman's Occupational Therapy*, 10th ed. by Crepeau, Cohn, and Schell

22. b. The amount of supervision in a particular setting is determined by the structure of the setting, amount of experience of the practitioner in that setting, and the acuity/needs of the patients. *Willard & Spackman's Occupational Therapy,* 10th ed. by Crepeau, Cohn, and Schell

23. c. The OTA conducted a treatment intervention that caused harm to the patient and the OT did not provide adequate supervision of the OTA or verify service competency in the area of hip precautions. Therefore, both professionals are liable. Any licensed healthcare professional who has a legal duty to care for a patient may be primarily liable for physical and mental injury incurred by the patient as a result of substandard care delivery. Clinical supervisors may incur liability indirectly or vicariously, even when they themselves do not cause the harm. *Willard & Spackman's Occupational Therapy*, 10th ed. by Crepeau, Cohn, and Schell, and *Promoting Legal Awareness in Physical and Occupational Therapy* by Scott

24. b. Medicare regulations permit occupational therapy services to continue after all other services have ended. *The Occupational Therapy Manager* by McCormack, Jaffe, and Goodman-Lavey

25. d. A prospective system pays a predetermined rate per episode (e.g., inpatient admission) based on an established scale. Medicare rates for inpatient hospitalization are based on diagnosis-related groups. *The Occupational Therapy Manager* by McCormack, Jaffe, and Goodman-Lavey

26. b. In capitation, a fixed amount is periodically paid to the provider for delivery of services for all persons covered under the contract or policy. There is no variation of the amount based on the number of person served. *The Occupational Therapy Manager* by McCormack, Jaffe, and Goodman-Lavey

27. c. Acute length of stay is usually <2 weeks; inpatient rehab is usually 2–4 weeks; home health may be longer but is rarely 5 days per week; skilled nursing facility length of stay varies with patient needs. *Willard & Spackman's Occupational Therapy,* 10th ed. by Crepeau, Cohn, and Schell

28. b. An indirect or operating cost is not related to the delivery of service but supports the general operation of the department. Salary and supply costs will vary depending on the amount and types of treatment provided. *The Occupational Therapy Manager* by McCormack, Jaffe, and Goodman-Lavey

29. b. Capital expenses must meet a minimum defined cost (typically $500 or $1000) and have an expected life of at least 3–5 years. The minimum dollar amount cannot be reached by

adding multiple items. *The Occupational Therapy Manager* by McCormack, Jaffe, and Goodman-Lavey

30. b. Profit margin is computed by taking profit (revenue − expenses) divided by total revenue. *The Occupational Therapy Manager* by McCormack, Jaffe, and Goodman-Lavey

31. a. 75% of 9 hours is 6.75 hour. She has already used 1.75 hours of nonproductive activity, leaving .5 hour. *The Occupational Therapy Manager* by McCormack, Jaffe, and Goodman-Lavey

32. a. The Accreditation Council for Occupational Therapy Education is the recognized body that accredits occupational and occupational therapy assistant programs. *The Occupational Therapy Manager* by McCormack, Jaffe, and Goodman-Lavey

33. d. Title control or trademark law protects the titles of OT and occupational therapy assistant but not specific occupational therapy treatments. Persons without the qualifications to perform occupational therapy can claim to offer those services. *The Occupational Therapy Manager* by McCormack, Jaffe, and Goodman-Lavey

34. b. Many states require completion of continuing competence or continuing education as part of license renewal. Certificates of moral character and proof of NBCOT certification are required for initial licensure, registration, or certification. *The Occupational Therapy Manager* by McCormack, Jaffe, and Goodman-Lavey

35. c. Most states mandate that all healthcare professionals report suspected abuse and neglect of vulnerable individuals. *Psychosocial Aspects of Health Care* by Drench

36. c. Ergonomic consulting is considered to be an emerging practice area by AOTA. Ergonomic consulting programs provide customers with expert, value-added ergonomic services to improve or continue the health and effectiveness of individuals in the workplace. *AOTA Emerging Practice Areas*

37. b. Writing a business plan allows aspiring entrepreneurs to describe the fundamental business concepts and provide critical information to decision makers, that is, lenders and investors. *Business Fundamentals for the Rehabilitation Professional* by Richmond and Powers

38. a. Controlling is the management function in which performance is measured against expectations and taking action to eliminate

obstacles to achieving organizational goals. An example of a control mechanism is productivity standards by measuring the output of an occupational therapy clinic or department. *Leading and Managing Occupational Therapy Services. An Evidence-Based Approach* by Braveman

39. b.   Outpatient service providers must match services specific to Current Procedural Terminology codes to ensure that services will be covered. Reimbursement fees are attached to each Current Procedural Terminology code. *The Occupational Therapy Manager* by McCormack, Jaffe, and Goodman-Lavey

40. a.   Effective communication by supervisors/managers involves communicating expectations, offering constructive criticisms, and expressing interest in an employee's professional growth. *The Occupational Therapy Manager* by McCormack, Jaffe, and Goodman-Lavey

41. d.   Advocacy skills include client advocacy, professional advocacy, advocacy with professional organizations, and advocacy with the healthcare environment. *Health Services Policy and Systems for Therapists* by Sandstrom, Lohman, and Bramble

42. b.   The purpose of regulating occupational therapy practice is to safeguard the public health, safety, and welfare; to protect the public from incompetent, unethical, or unauthorized persons; to ensure a high level of professional conduct on the part of occupational therapy practitioners; and to ensure the availability of high-quality occupational therapy services to people in need of those services. *Model Occupational Therapy Practice Act* by AOTA

43. a.   The relationship between management and leadership is that the role of a manager is to maintain stability, whereas a leader guides change and looks to the future. It has been suggested that whereas management is conservative and maintenance directed, leadership is innovative, change oriented, and informed by vision. *Leading and Managing Occupational Therapy Services. An Evidence-Based Approach* by Braveman

44. a.   Strategic planning within an organization provides the direction for that organization's mission and programs over a set period of time. *Leading and Managing Occupational Therapy Services. An Evidence-Based Approach* by Braveman

45. a. Part A Medicare is considered the hospital (inpatient) insurance benefit, whereas Part B Medicare is considered the supplementary medical insurance. *Health Services Policy and Systems for Therapists* by Sandstrom, Lohman, and Bramble

46. d. On the professional level, therapists advocate with peer professionals and with others, such as insurers. There are times in employment settings that OTs may identify misconduct in the way peer professionals deal with clients. Such matters should be reported to the appropriate agency (e.g., state licensure board) for review. *Health Services Policy and Systems for Therapists* by Sandstrom, Lohman, and Bramble

47. a. A business plan is the business concept's organizational tool and the marketing plan is the communication tool. In order to put together a successful business plan, one must develop marketing strategies. Conducting research on the targeted industry (i.e., healthcare) and the potential clients (target market) is the first step and provides input on ways to approach and identify those that will benefit from the program. *Business Fundamentals for the Rehabilitation Professional* by Richmond and Powers

48. d. A SWOT analysis is performed to analyze how effectively a business is operating relative to multiple factors, for example, patient population, the community, and the healthcare system. Issues that fall under the "threat" category are usually outside factors that are threatening the viability/sustainability of the business. *Business Fundamentals for the Rehabilitation Professional* by Richmond and Powers

49. c. Knowing the productivity requirement of 6 hours per day with a projected 24 hours of treatment per day, you can determine how many OTs are needed for each day by dividing how many daily units an OT can provide into the total units for that day. Therefore: 24 hours of patient treatment per day/6 hours productivity per OT = 4.0 FTEs. *The Occupational Therapy Manager* by McCormack, Jaffe, and Goodman-Lavey

50. a. The ADA requires employers to be inclusive of an individual who meets the job requirements of the employment position who, with or without reasonable accommodation, can perform the essential functions of the job. In order to determine what "reasonable accommodation" is, an employer must identify the essential and marginal functions of the job. *Leading and*

Managing Occupational Therapy Services. An Evidence-Based Approach by Braveman

51. a. Reasonable accommodation is a modification or an adjustment to a job or the work environment that will enable a qualified applicant or employee with a disability to participate in the application process or to perform the essential functions of the job. Reasonable accommodation includes adjustments to ensure that qualified person with a disability has rights and privileges of employment equal to those of nondisabled employees. Medication monitoring is not considered a reasonable accommodation. *Leading and Managing Occupational Therapy Services. An Evidence-Based Approach* by Braveman and *The Management of Musculoskeletal Disorders* by Sanders

52. d. According to the *OT Practice Framework* (AOTA, 2002), outcome assessment information is used to plan future actions with clients and to evaluate the service program (i.e., program evaluation).

53. a. The retention of valued employees is a major concern for occupational therapy managers and supervisors. Significant costs are associated with employee turnover, including recruitment expenses, lost revenue, and the need to train new employees. Retention of employees is no longer a primary function of human resources; rather the responsibility has shifted to line managers, for example, occupational therapy managers. An effective strategy to address high turnover related to limited growth opportunities is to involve the employees in work process design and offer growth and development opportunities. *Leading and Managing Occupational Therapy Services. An Evidence-Based Approach* by Braveman

54. c. The retention of valued employees is a major concern for occupational therapy managers and supervisors. Significant costs are associated with employee turnover, including recruitment expenses, lost revenue, and the need to train new employees. Retention of employees is no longer a primary function of human resources; rather the responsibility has shifted to line managers, for example, occupational therapy managers. An effective strategy to address high turnover related to pay inequities is to use market information to determine wage and benefit programs. *Leading and Managing Occupational Therapy Services. An Evidence-Based Approach* by Braveman

55. c. School-based occupational therapy is provided when the child needs support in the academic environment to perform

functional tasks to meet educational goals. *Occupational Therapy for Children* by Case-Smith

56. a. Approximately 95% of older Americans live in community settings, and health insurance companies promote this idea. The importance of place and its meaning, such as home, is receiving more focus than any other area being emphasized as a need for the elderly in the future. *Functional Performance in Older Adults* by Bonder and Wagner

57. b. Physical therapy and nursing are most likely to be concerned and involved with assessing the mobility skills of the client. *Functional Performance in Older Adults* by Bonder and Wagner

58. c. Acute care refers to short-term medical care provided during the acute phase of an illness or injury, when the symptoms are generally the most severe. The child will be admitted to acute care center this time and will need periodic hospitalization for issues relating to progressive illness. *Occupational Therapy for Children* by Case-Smith

59. a. Intervention for a school age child can best be facilitated through school-based services. The best course of action for transitioning to school from a rehabilitation unit is for the OT to set up at least one interagency meeting in which therapists share information about concerns, priorities, the results of interventions, and any accommodations that the child might need. *Occupational Therapy for Children* by Case-Smith

60. d. Under the program of special education, the child is eligible for related services to support special education, discipline-specific assessment as related to education, and an IEP. *Occupational Therapy for Children* by Case-Smith

61. a. A market analysis gathers information about the desires and needs of the target population or those who will be the recipient of the service, program, or product. *Leading and Managing Occupation Therapy Services* by Braveman

62. b. As defined in the Enforcement Procedures for Occupational Therapy Code of Ethics, a reprimand is "A formal expression of disapproval of conduct communicated privately by letter from the Chairperson of the EC that is nondisclosable and noncommunicative to other bodies (e.g., State Regulatory Boards, National Board for Certification in Occupational Therapy, etc)." *AOTA: Enforcement Procedures for Occupational Therapy Code of Ethics Document*

63. d. Veracity means truth. Principle 6 of the Code of Ethics addresses the fact that occupational therapy practitioners shall provide accurate information when representing the profession and "refrain from using or participating in the use of any form of communication that contains false, fraudulent, deceptive, or unfair statements or claims." *AOTA: Code of Ethics Document*

64. b. In ensuring confidentiality, the OT should "protect all privileged confidential forms of written, verbal, and electronic communication gained from educational, practice, research, and investigational activities unless otherwise mandated by local, state, or federal regulations." Written consent must be obtained from the client before releasing information. *AOTA: Code of Ethics Document*

65. a. Suspension is an action sometimes taken by the Ethics Commission that involves the removal of membership for a specified period of time. *AOTA: Enforcement Procedures for Occupational Therapy Code of Ethics Document*

66. a. A "Sua Sponte" complaint may be initiated by the Ethics Commissions when they are informed of a practitioner's ethical violation from a governmental body, certification or licensing body, public media, or other sources. *AOTA: Enforcement Procedures for Occupational Therapy Code of Ethics Document*

67. d. Service competency occurs when two practitioners performing the same procedure gain the same results. Service competency will need to be established between the OT and OTA or entry-level OT and supervisor so that these individuals master specific techniques, assessments, etc. *Clinical Competencies in Occupational Therapy* by Kief and Scheerer

68. b. The Family Educational Rights and Privacy Act was passed by Congress to allow parents and students access to educational records and confidentiality of the records from others. *Ethics in Rehabilitation* by Kornblau and Starling

69. d. In long term care facilities, the PPS uses Resource Utilization Grouping (RUG). Using an assessment tool called the Minimum Data Set (MDS) the OT, PT, SLP, and Nursing screens and assesses residents and categorizes them into a RUG category based on the number of minutes of therapy per week required to treat the resident. *The Occupational Therapy Manager* by McCormack, Jaffe, and Goodman-Lavey

70. b. SWOT Analysis begins with an internal and external environmental assessment of Strengths, Weaknesses, Opportunities, and Threats that can affect the organization or programs and then considers these factors in a strategic plan that is developed to help the organization reach its mission and vision. *The Occupational Therapy Manager* by McCormack, Jaffe, and Goodman-Lavey

71. b. In the Core Values and Attitude document, the specific core value that emphasizes the importance of valuing the inherent worth and uniqueness of each person is dignity. *Willard & Spackman's Occupational Therapyy,* 10th ed. by Crepeau, Cohn, and Schell

72. d. Informed consent refers to providing and sharing healthcare information to individuals so that they can make the best decisions about their treatment or healthcare. *Ethics in Rehabilitation: A Clinical Perspective* by Kornblau and Starling

73. a. Medicare will cover occupational therapy services if they are (1) prescribed by a physician according to a plan of care; (2) considered reasonable and necessary; and (3) performed by a qualified OT. *The Occupational Therapy Manager* by McCormack, Jaffe, and Goodman-Lavey

74. b. The Health Insurance Portability and Accountability Act (HIPAA) governs the interchange of healthcare information and financial and administrative data and protects the confidentiality of information about individual clients. *The Occupational Therapy Manager* by McCormack, Jaffe, and Goodman-Lavey

75. d. There are fours stages in the consultation process. In order of hierarchy, they are (1) initiation and clarification; (2) assessment and communication; (3) interactive problem solving; and (4) evaluation and clarification. *The Occupational Therapy Manager* by McCormack, Jaffe, and Goodman-Lavey

76. a. Memory impairments are normally the first deficits to be observed in persons with Alzheimer's disease. *Psychosocial Occupational Therapy: A Clinical Practice* by Cara and MacRae

77. c. A control group is compared to the experimental group. The control group may be treated in two ways: either receive no intervention or a different intervention than the experimental group. *Clinical Research in Occupational Therapy* by Stein and Cutler

78. a. The hypothesis is a statement of prediction. It hypothesizes the results of the study. *Clinical Research in Occupational Therapy* by Stein and Cutler

79. a. The occupational therapy process consist of three areas: the evaluation including the development of the occupational profile, the intervention (goal setting, intervention planning, intervention), and outcomes (the results of the intervention). *Applying the Occupational Therapy Practice Framework* by Skubik-Peplaski, Paris, Boyle, and Culpert

80. d. The "gold standard (p. 99)," for research evidence is randomized control trials in which subjects are randomly assigned to experimental or control groups. In descending order, the strongest to weakest level of evidence are demonstrated in randomized control trials, cohort studies, cross-sectional surveys, and case studies, respectively. *Evidence-Based Rehabilitation: A Guide to Practice* by Law

81. c. Process evaluation provides an ongoing account of what is occurring in a program. It examines processes and the internal mechanisms on how the program is working, whereas a summative evaluation focuses on outcomes and results of a program. *Occupational Therapy in Community-Based Practice* by Scaffa

82. c. It is crucial to take the patient's feelings into consideration when you have to let them know that it is unethical to accept gifts. By explaining the situation and acknowledging the gesture you are more likely to avoid offending the patient. *Mental Health Concepts and Techniques for the Occupational Therapy Assistant* by Early

83. b. There are five steps to the evidence-based practice clinical reasoning and problem solving process: 1) formulate the question; 2) search and sort the evidence; 3) critically appraise the evidence; 4) apply to practice (accept or reject results); and 5) conduct self -assessment. *Mental Health Concepts and Techniques for the Occupational Therapy Assistant* by Early

84. a. First discussed in the literature 1987 and then again in 1989, this model was conceptualized to explain the exacerbation and remission of symptoms observed in schizophrenic patients who were living in the community. *Occupational Therapy in Community-Based Practice Settings* by Scaffa

85. c. Our scope of practice does not include diagnosing or prescribing medications. We need a physician's order to treat and currently lack recognition as "qualified mental health providers" (QMHP) in many states. *AOTA*

86. b. In community settings, OTs fulfill a clinical role but also often serve as the case manager for many of the clients that they see. *Occupational Therapy in Community-Based Practice Settings* by Scaffa

87. d. Occupational therapy is a holistic practice that addresses the physical, psychosocial, and spiritual needs of all patients. No specialty certification is currently required. *Mental Health Concepts and Techniques for the Occupational Therapy Assistant* by Early

88. a. Families can be a great source of support for patients in treatment. *Proactive Approaches in Psychosocial Occupational Therapy* by Fleming

89. c. Even the sickest patient may be able to benefit from occupational therapy services. OTs are exceptional at adapting the intervention to meet the client's present needs. *Mental Health Concepts and Techniques for the Occupational Therapy Assistant* by Early

90. a. It is crucial that information that may influence treatment remains confidential and is shared with no one except the team that is treating the patient. If so desired, the patient may choose to share the information about being sexually abused with others. However, sharing private information should be the individual's choice. *Mental Health Concepts and Techniques for the Occupational Therapy Assistant* by Early

91. a. The symptoms include lip smacking, tongue protrusion, and so forth and even with discontinuance of the medication, they may never go away. *Psychopathology and Function* by Bonder

92. c. In 2002, Medicare implemented a prospective payment system for inpatient rehabilitation facilities and hospitals that classified patients into categories called case mixed groups (CMGs). CMGs are derived from scores on patient assessment instruments which measure person functional motor and cognitive abilities. *The Occupational Therapy Manager* by McCormack, Jaffe, and Goodman-Lavey

93. c. OTs are trained to address the occupational performance needs of patients, including the area of sexual dysfunction. It is also beneficial that additional referrals be made to specialists to ensure that the patient gets the highest quality of care. *Conditions in Occupational Therapy: Effects on Occupational Performance* by Hansen

94. a. In skilled nursing facilities, a resident assessment instrument called the Minimum Data Set is used as a screening, clinical, and functional status assessment that classifies clients into resource utilization groups. Prospective payment rates are then established based on the client's status according to the Minimum Data Set. *Conditions in Occupational Therapy: Effect on Occupational Performance* by Hansen

95. a. OTs serve as consultants to self-help groups, which are organized and lead by the individual members whose lives are directly impacted by the condition. *Mental Health Concepts and Techniques for the Occupational Therapy Assistant* by Early and *DSM-IV-TR* by the American Psychiatric Association

96. b. If the pattern of behavior involving disregard for the rights of others continues into adulthood the person will likely be diagnosed with antisocial personality disorder. *DSM-IV-TR* by the American Psychiatric Association

97. d. The student is unable to name or legibly write letters and numbers because of delayed visual motor skills. A student's IEP must include a statement of the child's present levels of performance, reflecting the child's ability to perform in the curriculum. *Occupational Therapy for Children* by Case-Smith

98. a. The following are included within the definition of related services: speech-language pathology and audiology services; psychological services; physical and occupational therapy; recreation, including therapeutic recreation; assistive technology devices and services; counseling services, including rehabilitation counseling; orientation and mobility services; medical services for diagnostic or evaluation purposes; school health services; social work services in schools; parent counseling and training; and transportation. *OT Services for Children and Youth Under the IDEA*

99. d. Although federal funding provides part of the cost of special education, IDEA encourages states to establish interagency agreements or other arrangements to seek funding from noneducational public agencies such as private insurance and state Medicaid agencies. Students are entitled to receive services

at no cost to themselves or their families. NICHCY Related Services News Digest 16, 2nd Edition, 2001 (http://www.nichcy.org/pubs/newsdig/nd16txt.htm)

100. d. The OT has overall responsibility for implementing intervention. The OTA is responsible for being knowledgeable about student goals as well as selecting, implementing, and modifying therapeutic activities; however, the OT maintains overall responsibility for implementing intervention. *AOTA Guidelines for Supervision, Roles, and Responsibilities During the Delivery of Occupational Therapy Services*

101. d. C.F.R. 300.344 and 300.346–347 identifies required components of an IEP as well as IEP team members. *OT Services for Children and Youth Under IDEA* by AOTA

102. a. When transitioning from one role to another, educational preparation is essential to assume the new duties. Individuals changing roles will typically require close supervision as they learn new tasks and routines. *AOTA Official Documents: Occupational Therapy Roles*

103. b. Routine supervision is defined as direct contact at least every 2 weeks at the place of employment, with interim supervision occurring by telephone or through written communication. *AOTA Official Documents: Occupational Therapy Roles*

104. b. The major focus of a practitioner functioning at the intermediate level is to master basic roles with increased independence and to be able to respond based on previous experience. Progression through the roles of entry level (the development of skills), intermediate (mastery of role), and advance (specialization and refined skills) is based on the accumulation of higher level skills through experience, education, and professional development. *AOTA Official Documents: Occupational Therapy Roles*

105. b. Universal design relate to features of the built environment that enhance optimal function and convenience for everyone regardless of disability. *Occupational Therapy for Physical Dysfunction* by Trombly and Radomski

106. c. Consultation is an interactive process of helping others solve existing or potential problems by identifying and analyzing issues and developing strategies to solve problems and to prevent future problems. *The Occupational Therapy Manager* by McCormack, Jaffe, and Goodman-Lavey

Selected Bibliography and Suggested Reading

American Occupational Therapy Association: Occupational therapy practice framework: domain and process. *Am J Occup Ther* 56:609–39, 2002.

American Occupational Therapy Association: Standards of practice for occupational therapy. *Am J Occup Ther* 59:663–5, 2005.

American Occupational Therapy Association: Statement of occupational therapy referral. *Am J Occup Ther* 48:1034, 1994.

American Occupational Therapy Association: *Occupational therapy services for children and youth under the Individuals with Disabilities Education Act (IDEA)*, Bethesda, Md, 1999, AOTA Press.

American Occupational Therapy Association: Scope of practice, *Am J Occup Ther* 58:673–7, 2004

American Occupational Therapy Association: *Work: principles and practice,* (self-paced clinical course), Bethesda, Md, 2000, AOTA Press.

American Occupational Therapy Association: Occupational therapy code of ethics (2005), *Am J Occup Ther* 59:639–42, 2005.

American Occupational Therapy Association: *Guidelines for documentation of occupational therapy*, Bethesda, Md, 2003, AOTA Press.

Acquaviva JD: *Effective documentation for occupational therapy,* ed 2, Bethesda, Md, 1998, AOTA Press.

American Psychiatric Association: *Diagnostic and statistical manual of mental disorders, fourth edition, text revision (DSM-IV-TR)*, Arlington, Va, 2000, American Psychiatric Association.

Bloom M, Fischer J, Orme JG: *Evaluating practice: guidelines for the accountable professional*, ed 2, Boston, Mass, 1998, Allyn & Bacon.

Bonder B, Wagner M: *Functional performance in older adults,* Philadelphia, Pa, 2001, F.A. Davis.

Bonder BR: *Psychpathology and function,* ed 2, Thorofare, NJ, 1995, SLACK, Incorporated.

Borcherding S, Kappel C: *The OTA's guide to writing SOAP notes*, Thorofare, NJ, 2002, SLACK, Incorporated.

Braveman B: *Leading and managing occupational therapy services. An evidence-based approach,* Philadelphia, Pa, 2006, F.A. Davis.

Brayman SJ, Clark GF, DeLany JV, et al, for the American Occupational Therapy Association Commission on Practice: Guidelines for supervision, roles, and responsibilities during the delivery of occupational therapy services (2004), *Am J Occup Ther* 58:663–7, 2004.

Brownson RC, Baker EA, Left TL, et al: *Evidence-based public health*, Oxford, 2003, Oxford University Press.

Bundy AC, Lane SJ, Murray EA, eds: *Sensory integration: theory and practice,* ed 2, Philadelphia, Pa, 2002, F.A. Davis.

Burke SL, Higgins JP, McClinton MA, et al, eds: *Upper extremity rehabilitation: a practical guide,* St. Louis, Mo, 2006, Elsevier.

Cara E, MacRae A, eds: *Psychosocial occupational therapy: a clinical practice*, Clifton Park, NY, 2005, Thomson Delmar Learning.

Case-Smith J: *Occupational therapy for children,* ed 5, St. Louis, 2005, Mosby.

Case-Smith J, ed: *Pediatric occupational therapy and early intervention,* ed 2, Woburn, Mass, 1997, Butterworth-Heinemann.

Christiansen CH, Matuska, KM, eds: *Ways of living: adaptive strategies for special needs,* ed 3, Bethesda, Md, 2004, AOTA Press.

Christiansen CH, Baum C: *Occupational therapy: enabling function and well-being,* ed 2, Thorofare, NJ, 1997, SLACK, Incorporated.

Christiansen CH, Townsend EA, eds: *Introduction to occupation: the art and science of living,* Upper Saddle River, NJ, 2004, Prentice Hall.

Christiansen CH, Baum C, eds: *Occupational therapy: overcoming human performance deficits,* Thorofare, NJ, 1991, SLACK, Incorporated.

Cole MB: *Group dynamics in occupational therapy,* ed 3, Thorofare, NJ, 2005, SLACK, Incorporated.

Cook AM, Hussey SM: *Assistive technologies: principles and practice,* ed 2, St. Louis, Mo, 2002, Mosby.

Coppard B, Lohman H: *Introduction to splinting: a clinical reasoning and problem solving approach,* ed 2, St. Louis, Mo, 2001, Mosby.

Clarkson HM: *Musculoskeletal assessment,* ed 2, Philadelphia, Pa, 2000, Lippincott Williams & Wilkins.

Crepeau EB, Cohn ES, Schell BAB, eds: *Willard and Spackman's occupational therapy,* ed 10, Philadelphia, Pa, 2003, Lippincott Williams & Wilkins.

Cronin A, Mandich M: *Human development and performance: throughout the lifespan,* New York, NY, 2005, Thomson Delmar Learning.

Denzin NK, Lincoln YS: *Handbook of qualitative research,* ed 2, Thousand Oaks, Calif, 2000, Sage.

Depoy E, Gilson S: *Evaluation practice: thinking and action principles for social work practice,* Belmont, Calif, 2003, Wadsworth

DePoy E, Gitlin L: *Introduction to research: understanding and applying multiple strategies,* ed 3, St. Louis, Mo, 2005, Mosby.

Dunn W: *Best practice in occupational therapy in community service with children and families,* Thorofare, NJ, 2000, SLACK, Incorporated.

Early MB: *Mental health concepts and techniques for the occupational therapy assistant,* ed 2, New York, NY, 1993, Raven Press.

Weiss S, Falkenstein N: *Hand rehabilitation: a quick reference guide and review,* ed 2, St. Louis, Mo, 2005, Mosby.

Finlay L: *The practice of psychosocial occupational therapy,* ed 3, Cheltenham, 2004, Nelson Thornes.

Finnie N: *Handling the young child with cerebral palsy at home,* ed 3, Woburn, Mass, 1997, Butterworth-Heinemann.

Fitzpatrick JL, Sanders JR, Worthen BR: *Program evaluation: alternative approaches and practical guidelines,* ed 3, Boston, Mass, 2003, Allyn & Bacon.

Fleming Cottrell RP: *Proactive approaches in psychosocial occupational therapy,* Thorofare, NJ, 2000, SLACK, Incorporated.

Gillen G, Burkhardt A, eds: *Stroke rehabilitation: a function-based approach,* ed 2, St. Louis, Mo, 2004, Elsevier Mosby.

Grinell RM: *Social work research and evaluation,* ed 6, Itasca, Ill, 2001, Peacock.

Hansen RA, Atchison B, eds: *Conditions in occupational therapy: effect on occupational performance,* ed 2, Baltimore, Md, 2000, Lippincott Williams & Wilkins.

Hemphill-Pearson BJ, ed: *Assessments in occupational therapy mental health: an integrative approach,* Thorofare, NJ, 1999, SLACK, Incorporated.

Henderson A, Pehoski C, eds: *Hand function in the child: foundations for remediation,* St. Louis, Mo, 1995, Mosby.

Hinojosa J, Kramer P: *Occupational therapy evaluation: obtaining and interpreting data,* Bethesda, Md, 1998, AOTA Press.

Hislop HJ, Montgomery J: *Daniels and Worthingham's muscle testing,* ed 7, Philadelphia, Pa, 2002, W.B. Saunders.

Jacobs K, ed: *Ergonomics for therapists*, ed 2, Boston, Mass, 1999, Butterworth-Heinemann.

Johnstone B, Stonnington H, Stonnington HH, eds: *Rehabilitation of neuropsychological disorders: a practical guide for rehabilitation professionals and family members,* Brighton, NY, 2001, Psychology Press.

Katz N, ed: *Occupation and cognition across the lifespan: models for intervention in occupational therapy*, Bethesda, Md, 2005, AOTA Press.

Kettenbach G: *Writing SOAP notes*, ed 3, Philadelphia, Pa, 2004, F.A. Davis.

Kief CA, Scheerer CR: *Clinical competencies in occupational therapy*, Upper Saddle River, NJ, 2001, Prentice Hall.

Kielhofner G, ed: *A model of human occupation*, Baltimore, Md, 2002, Willliam & Wilkins.

Kielhofner G, ed: *Conceptual foundations of occupational therapy*, ed 3, Philadelphia, Pa, 2004, F.A. Davis.

Kornblau BL, Jacobs K, eds: *Work: principles and practice*, Bethesda, Md, 2000, AOTA Press.

Kornblau BL, Starling SP: *Ethics in rehabilitation: a clinical perspective*, Thorofare, NJ, 2000, SLACK, Incorporated.

Kramer P, Hinojosa J, Royeen CB, eds: *Perspectives in human occupation: participation in life*, Baltimore, Md, 2003, Lippincott Williams & Wilkins.

Kramer P, Hinojosa J: *Frames of reference for pediatric occupational therapy,* Baltimore, Md, 1999, Lippincott Williams & Wilkins

Law M, Baum CM, Baptiste S: *Occupation-based practice: fostering performance and participation*, Thorofare, NJ, 2002, SLACK, Incorporated.

Law MC, Baptiste S, Carswell A, et al: *The Canadian occupational performance measure*, Ottawa, Ontario, 1998, CAOT Publications.

Law MC, ed: *Evidence-based rehabilitation: a guide to practice*, Thorofare, NJ, 2002, SLACK, Incorporated.

Lewis CB, ed: *Aging: the health care challenge: an interdisciplinary approach to assessment and rehabilitation management of the elderly*, ed 4, Philadelphia, Pa, 2002, F.A. Davis.

Lundy-Ekman L: *Neuroscience. Fundamentals for rehabilitation*, ed 2, Philadelphia, Pa, 2002, W.B. Saunders

McCormack GL, Jaffe EG, Goodman-Lavey M, eds: *The occupational therapy manager*, ed 4, Bethseda, Md, 2003, AOTA Press.

Parham LD, Fazio LS, eds: *Play in occupational therapy for children*, St. Louis, Mo, 1997, Mosby.

Patton MQ: *Qualitative research and evaluation methods*, Thousand Oaks, Calif, 2001, Sage.

Pedretti L, Early MB: *Occupational therapy: practice skills for physical dysfunction*, ed 5, St. Louis, 2001, Mosby.

Pendleton H, Schultz-Krohn W, eds: *Pedretti's occupational therapy: practice skills for physical dysfunction,* ed 6, St. Louis, Mo, 2006, Mosby.

Punwar A, Peloquin S: *Occupational therapy, principles & practice*, ed 3, Philadelphia, Pa, 2000, Lippincott Williams & Wilkins.

Purtilo R: *Ethical dimensions in the health professions,* ed 4, Philadelphia, Pa, 2005, W.B. Saunders.

Reed KL, Sanderson SR: *Concepts of occupational therapy,* ed 4, Philadelphia, Pa, 1999, Lippincott Williams & Wilkins

Reed KL: *Quick reference to occupational therapy*, ed 2, Philadelphia, Pa, 2000, Lippincott Williams & Wilkins

Rosen A: *Evidence-based social work practice: challenges and promises*, Address at the Society for Social Work and Research, 2002, San Diego, Calif.

Royeen M, Crabtree JL, eds: *Culture in rehabilitation: from competency to proficiency*, Upper Saddle River, NJ, 2006, Pearson/Prentice Hall.

Royse D, Thyer B, Padgett DK, et al: *Program evaluation: an introduction*, Belmont, Calif, 2000, Wadsworth.

Sackett DL, Straus SE, Richardson WS, et al: *Evidence-based medicine: how to practice and teach EBM*, ed 2, New York, NY, 2000, Churchill Livingstone.

Sanders MJ, ed: *Ergonomics and the management of musculoskeletal disorders,* ed 2, St. Louis, Mo, 2004, Butterworth-Heinemann.

Sames KM: *Documenting occupational therapy practice*, Upper Saddle River, NJ, 2005, Pearson/Prentice Hall.

Scaffa ME: *Occupational therapy in community-based practice settings*, Philadelphia, Pa, 2001, F.A. Davis.

Scott R: *Professional ethics: a guide for rehabilitation professionals*, St. Louis, Mo, 1998, Mosby.

Skubik-Peplaski C, Paris C, Collins Boyle DR, Culpert A: *Applying the occupational therapy practice framework: The Cardinal Hill occupational participation process,* Bethesda, Md, 2006, AOTA Press.

Sine R, Liss SE, Roush RE, et al: Basic rehabilitation techniques: a self-instructional guide, ed 4, New York, NY, 2000, Aspen Publishers, Inc.

Sladyk K, Ryan SE, eds: *Ryan's occupational therapy assistant: principles, practice issues, and techniques,* ed 4, Thorofare, NJ, 2005, SLACK, Incorporated.

Sladyk K, ed: *The successful occupational therapy fieldwork student*, Thorofare, NJ, 2002, SLACK, Incorporated.

Sabonis-Chafee B, Hussey SM: *Introduction to occupational therapy,* ed 2, St. Louis, Mo, 1998, Mosby.

Solomon A, Jacobs K, eds: *Management skills for the occupational therapy assistant*, Thorofare NJ, 2003, SLACK, Incorporated.

Solomon J, O'Brien J, eds: *Pediatric skills for occupational therapy assistants,* St. Louis, Mo, 2006, Mosby.

Sonnert G: *Ivory bridges: connecting science and society*, Cambridge, Mass, 2002, MIT Press.

Steier F: *Research and reflexivity*, Newbury Park, Calif, 1991, Sage.

Stein F, Cutler S, eds: *Clinical research in allied health and special education,* ed 3, San Diego, Calif, 1996, Singular Press.

Stein F, Cutler S: *Psychosocial occupational therapy: a holistic approach*, San Diego, Calif, 1998, Singular Press.

Thyer B: *The handbook of social work research methods*, Thousand Oaks, Calif, 2001, Sage.

Trombly CA, Radomski MV: *Occupational therapy for physical dysfunction*, ed 5, Baltimore, Md, 2002, Lippincott Williams & Wilkins.

Unrau YA, Gabor PA, Grinnell RM: *Evaluation in the human services*, Itasca, Ill, 2001, Peacock.

Van Dusen J, Brunt D, eds: *Assessment in occupational therapy and physical therapy*, Philadelphia, Pa, 1997, W.B. Saunders.

World Health Organization: *International classification of functioning, disability and health (ICF)*, Geneva, Switzerland, 2001, WHO.

Yin R: *Case study research: design and methods*, ed 2, Thousand Oaks, Calif, 2003, Sage.

Youngstrom MJ: The occupational therapy practice framework: the evolution of our professional language, *Am J Occup Ther* 56:607–8, 2002.

Zoltan B: *Vision, perception and cognition*, ed 3, Thorofare, NJ, 1996, SLACK, Incorporated.

Index

A

Abductor pollicis longus tendon, in
   de Quervain's tenosynovitis, 34, 84
Accommodation, 11, 66–67
Accountability, 279–280, 296
Accreditation, of occupational therapy
   education programs
Accreditation Council for
   Occupational Therapy Education,
   266, 286
Acquired immunodeficiency
   syndrome (AIDS) patients,
   59, 102
Acquisition, in learning, 167, 223
Acting out, 204, 250
Active range of motion, evaluation of,
   20, 75
Active range-of-motion exercises, for
   fracture patients, 19, 74
Activities, grading of. *See* Grading, of
   activities
Activities of daily living (ADL).
      See also Instrumental activities of
      daily living (IADL)
   deficits in
      in fibromyalgia patients, 127–128,
         153
      in hemiplegia patients, 182, 235
      progressive mobilization programs
         for, 177, 231
      in pulmonary disease patients,
         177, 210, 232, 254–255
      in spinal cord injury patients,
         20–21, 76
   efficiency of, 32, 83
   evaluation of, in cerebrovascular
      accident patients, 41–42, 89–90
Activities of daily living practice,
   202–203, 249–250

Activity analysis, 117, 146
Activity demands, 33, 83
Acute care, 271, 290
Adaptation, 162, 218
   as compensatory cognitive
      strategy, 130, 155
   components of, 11, 66–67
   postural, 57, 101
Adapted techniques, for hemiplegia
   patients, 182, 235–236
Adaptive motor response
   development, 190, 241
Adaptive responses
   definition of, 183, 236
   Sensory Integration Theory of,
      41, 89
Adaptive techniques
   for cerebrovascular accident patients,
      192–193, 242
   for visual acuity deficit patients, 192,
      242
Administration and service
   management, 8, 259–296
Administrative controls, ergonomic,
   186, 238
Adolescent Role Assessment, 48, 95
Adolescents
   acting out by, 204, 250
   anger management in, 213, 256
   conduct disorder in, 48, 95,
      134–135, 157
   maladaptive behavior in, 134, 157
   role performance evaluation of, 48, 95
   transition goals and services for, 125,
      151
   wheelchair use by, 116, 145
Adult day care, 109, 140
Advice giving, by occupational
   therapists, 49, 95

Touro College
OCCUPATIONAL THERAPY PROGRAM
1700 Union Boulevard
Bay Shore, NY 11706

WITHDRAWN